Edward Smith

Health

A Handbook for Households and Schools

Edward Smith

Health

A Handbook for Households and Schools

ISBN/EAN: 9783337404512

Printed in Europe, USA, Canada, Australia, Japan

Cover: Foto ©Paul-Georg Meister /pixelio.de

More available books at **www.hansebooks.com**

HEALTH

HEALTH:

A HANDBOOK FOR HOUSEHOLDS AND SCHOOLS.

BY

EDWARD SMITH, M.D., F.R.S.,

LL. B. (UNIV. OF LOND.),

FELLOW OF THE ROYAL COLLEGE OF PHYSICIANS OF LONDON AND OF THE ROYAL COLLEGE OF SURGEONS OF ENGLAND; INSPECTOR AND ASSISTANT MEDICAL OFFICER FOR POOR-LAW PURPOSES OF THE LOCAL GOVERNMENT BOARD; LATELY ASSISTANT PHYSICIAN TO THE HOSPITAL FOR CONSUMPTION, BROMPTON; CORRESPONDING MEMBER OF THE ACADEMY OF SCIENCES, MONTPELLIER, AND OF THE NATURAL HISTORY SOCIETY OF MONTREAL, ETC., ETC.

PREFACE.

Having been requested by the Publishers to write a small work on the subject of Health, which might be useful to the elder scholars in schools and to the public generally, I have done so in the hope that it may supply a want of prime magnitude. The limited size of the work, as well as the somewhat youthful persons to whom it is chiefly addressed, have rendered it as difficult as necessary to make a selection of materials, and to use very plain and simple language. I hope the subjects introduced will be deemed worthy of careful consideration, and that the familiar style of writing will not be unacceptable to any class of readers. Should any portion, as for example the chapter on atmospheric conditions, be found too far advanced for the attainments of young persons, the reading of it may be deferred for a time; but it is hoped that none is beyond the comprehension of adults in the masses of the people. Should it be found to be a useful addition to a higher class school series, I shall hope that the instruction may not be limited to this generation, but will be handed down to the children of the next.

EDWARD SMITH.

140, *Harley Street*,
    January, 1874.

CONTENTS.

CHAP.		PAGE
	PREFACE	v
	INTRODUCTORY	1
I.	SOLID FOODS:—	
	Sugar	5
	Honey	7
	Fat	8
	Starch	12
	Flour	14
	Dried Peas, Beans, and Lentils. . . .	16
	Bread	17
	Rice, Sago, Arrowroot, and Tapioca . . .	20
	Fresh Vegetables	23
	Butchers' Meat	28
	Uncooked Meat	32
	Offal	33
	Gelatin and Isinglass	34
	Bacon	35
	Poultry and Game	36
	Cheese	37
	Fish	38
	Eggs	39
II.	LIQUID FOODS:—	
	Milk	41
	Water	44
	Tea and Coffee	48
	Beer, Wine, and Spirits	53
III.	GENERAL QUESTIONS RELATING TO FOOD:—	
	Digestibility of Solid Foods	56
	Condiments	58

CHAP.		PAGE
	Poisonous Substances sometimes Eaten	59
	Tobacco	60
	Hints about Cooking	62
IV.	CLOTHING	70
V.	MOVEMENTS OF THE BODY:—	
	Exertion	74
	Occupation	77
	Recreation	80
	Gymnastics	82
VI.	REST AND SLEEP	95
VII.	CLEANLINESS AND BATHING	104
VIII.	DWELLINGS:—	
	Houses	109
	Ventilation	116
IX.	SKETCH OF PHYSIOLOGY	120
X.	ATMOSPHERIC CONDITIONS:—	
	Elements of the Atmosphere	136
	Pressure	142
	Moisture	143
	Electricity	146
	Light	147
XI.	THE MIND AND MENTAL WORK	150
XII.	THE SPECIAL SENSES:—	
	The Eye	155
	Ophthalmia in Schools	161
	The Ear	164
	The Nose	170
	Stuttering	170
XIII.	GENERAL REMARKS ON PERSONAL CONDUCT AND HEALTH	172
XIV.	THE SICK-ROOM:—	
	Contagious Diseases	179
	Colds, Coughs, Bronchitis, and Asthma	181
	Rheumatism	190
	Headache, &c.	192

LIST OF ILLUSTRATIONS.

FIG.		PAGE
1.	Fat Cells in Man	9
2 & 3.	Other Fat Cells	9
4.	Fat Cells of the Cocoa Nut	10
5.	Globules of Oil in Cream and Milk	10
6.	Starch Cells of many Plants	13
7.	Yeast Cells	16
8.	Section of Healthy Potato	25
9.	„ Diseased Potato	25
10.	„ „ „	26
11.	Strawberry Cells	26
12.	Muscular Fibre	28
13.	A Cistern Filter	46
14 to 34.	Illustrations of Gymnastic Exercises	86 to 94
35.	Section of the Heart	123
36.	Scheme of the Circulation	124
37.	Circulation in the Frog's Foot	125
38.	Circulation in the India-Rubber Plant	126
39.	Blood Corpuscles of numerous Animals	126
40.	The Lungs	127
41.	Section of the Skin	134
42.	Stomata or Mouths of Plants	140
43.	The Iris in the Eye	156
44.	Section of the Eye	158
45.	Section of the Ear	166
46.	Ossicles or Little Bones of the Ear	167
47.	The Cochlea of the Ear	168
48.	The Labyrinth of the Ear	169

HEALTH.

INTRODUCTORY.

AFTER ages of apathy, the people of this country have begun to recognise the fact that the mortality amongst us is excessive, and should be diminished. We now see in sickness the cause as well as the fruit of poverty, and in a low tone of health the antecedent of sickness, and are convinced that the evil may be ameliorated. This conviction is no doubt a pledge of better things; for, if we would lessen disease and mortality, we must remove or lessen their causes, and to do so we must inquire into them and devise suitable remedies. We have now arrived at a period when it has become even fashionable to speak of the origin of the most contagious diseases as due to preventible causes, and may therefore be presumed to have passed the shifting sands of mere theory and speculation, and to have placed our feet on the firm ground of ascertained facts.

Acting on this truth, great efforts are now put forth to remove such unsanitary conditions as may affect masses of the people, as defective drainage, accumulations of filth, overcrowded rooms, ill-ventilated workshops, and injurious trades, and to provide a supply of pure air and water, all of which tend both to prevent the occurrence of some epidemic diseases affecting many at the same moment, and to elevate the tone of health of individuals. Legislation is active, and official persons abound in every locality whose duty it is to enforce the law, and all that can be done *for* a people makes satisfactory progress.

The next and yet more difficult and important step is to bring about that which can be done *by* the people. Until those for whom we legislate are well informed on the subject of legislation, the progress, if sure, will be slow; but let us so enlighten the masses of the people that they shall individually appreciate the benefits to be conferred, and willingly assist, and success will be rapidly attained.

Sanitary knowledge is still almost restricted to the few who may teach and govern, and has not made many converts among the labouring men and their wives, who, with their children, furnish the chief part of the poverty, sickness, and mortality of the country—or, in other words, are the chief victims of unsanitary influences. Yet the beginning of better things appears in tracts and lectures on health, and in the influence of a certain number of persons of both sexes in numerous localities.

The most hopeful effort is, however, that which seeks to instil sanitary knowledge into the minds of the young, at the same time that they acquire the information which is to aid them in performing the active duties of life, and to show that however valuable the latter may be to ensure an income, the former is yet more useful, in preventing sickness and death. When, at the same time, the precepts thus inculcated are reduced to practice, we may look for a generation of men and women who will enjoy a higher degree of health and longer life than ourselves, and who will increase and hand down their knowledge to their children.

Such is the aim of the present work. It is intended to inform the mind on the subjects involved in the word Health, to show how health may be retained and ill-health avoided, and to add to the pleasure and usefulness of life. It addresses itself primarily to the young of both sexes, and although it necessarily embraces subjects of some difficulty to them, it is made less difficult by the omission of technical terms, and the use of plain language and simple statements. Hence, if read at school or by the fireside, its statements will be readily explained, and all that is valuable may be committed to memory.

But it is equally written for those of more advanced age, whose minds have not been specially directed to the subject, and it will, it is hoped, afford information to both the poor and rich members of the community.

A moment's reflection will show how wide is the subject of health, for it not only embraces a knowledge of the structures and functions of the body, but of all the influences which act upon it from without. Nothing is too great to be included or too small to be excluded by it. Hence a new difficulty arises, that of determining what shall be introduced and what withheld, and how much each subject may be discussed; for if the subject be so vast, what proportion of it can be compressed into a very small book? This would be treated differently by different authors, as each formed his estimate of the relative importance of the subjects to those whom he desired to instruct, and according to his own taste and knowledge in selecting and treating them. I can, therefore, hope only to have exercised a discretion which may not be very unwise, and, with whatever ability I possess, to have treated the subjects truthfully and simply.

With the subjects selected, it matters, perhaps, little as to the order in which they shall be treated, and yet some regard must be had to the limited knowledge and undeveloped faculties of the young, and the advantage of gaining, rather than of repelling, their attention. Hence, whilst it would, doubtless, be more logical first to explain the structure and action of the body, and the properties of the atmosphere which surrounds it, and then to proceed to other minute details, it may be asserted that the children of this country would fail to understand it, and would grow weary of the subject. It seems desirable to begin with a short account of foods, since they are familiar, and of daily use and observation, whilst they have an influence over health second to none, and to defer the more scientific and abstruse questions to the end of the volume, in the hope that, on arriving at them, the mind of the reader will be better prepared for their consideration and apprehension.

CHAPTER I.

SOLID FOODS.

Foods are not eaten indiscriminately, but carefully selected according to their qualities, so that some are popularly known to be stronger than others, and to have a special fitness for certain seasons or kinds of work. This knowledge may be very general, but it is not the less real; and the duty of science is to render it more precise by careful researches, and to explain the reasons for the course which experience has dictated. This has led to a division of foods according to their action or chemical composition, and we are now taught that they act in two ways, viz., by warming and sustaining the body. But all foods do not effect both objects, so that some are said to produce heat and others to repair waste. Thus sugar, fat, and starch make heat only, whilst nearly all other foods both produce heat and repair waste. We will shortly describe the principal foods of both classes.

SUGAR.

Sugar is found in nearly all foods, but particularly in fruits, and is collected in large quantities from the juices of many plants, as the sugar-cane, sugar-maple, and beetroot. It is obtained in crystals, mixed with a little treacle in moist sugar, but pure and made white by purification in loaf sugar. The larger the crystals and the less the treacle, the purer is the moist sugar, whilst the whiter and harder the loaf sugar the better is the quality.

That part of the juice in the sugar-cane which does not form crystals but remains a thick fluid, is called treacle, and, although very sweet, is less pure than sugar. When sugar is being purified so as to make loaf sugar, the treacle runs out of it and is called golden syrup, and is purer, although perhaps less sweet, than treacle from the cane juice.

There is also much sugar in milk, which is obtained in crystals, but it is more costly, and does not sweeten so well, as cane-sugar.

There are, therefore, three kinds of separated sugar in actual use,—viz., cane sugar, fruit sugar, and milk sugar, but the first is much more abundant than both the others.

Sugar is a valuable and universal food, and one by which other foods are made more palatable, and their nutritious qualities increased, but it is possible to eat it in excess. Thus, when it is added in a large quantity to milk for infants, it lessens the proportion of that part which repairs the body, and thereby tends to make the child unduly fat, whilst at the same time it destroys the relish for foods which are not so sweet. It is not taken alone, as a necessary food, but as a luxury, and is very liable to cause indigestion and bilious attacks. Hence, although so agreeable and useful, it should be eaten with foods in moderation, and the quantity may be reduced to a very low point without serious consequences. It is eaten in much larger proportion by the young than the old, and in hot than in cold countries, but usually from two to four ounces are eaten daily in our foods.

It is interesting to know the quantity which is usually found in foods, and it is shown in the following table.

Table No. 1.

Number of pounds of sugar which are found in 100 pounds of the following foods : *—

	lbs.
Rice and Indian meal	0·4
Peas	2·0
Turnips	2·1
Cream	2·8
Potatoes	3·2
Bread	3·6
Rye meal	3·7
Wheat flour	4·2
Barley meal	4·9
New milk	5·2
Oatmeal and Skim Milk	5·4
Parsnips	5·8
Butter Milk	6·4
Beer and Porter	8·7
Treacle	77·0
Moist Sugar	95·0

HONEY.

The chief food-ingredient in honey is sugar, which corresponds in character with fruit sugar. It is collected from flowers, where it is already formed, and is not produced by the bees. It has a peculiar flavour, which is also derived from flowers, and in some instances has been poisonous; but, speaking generally, it is a very agreeable and useful food. The collection of honey may be effected at a very small cost and greatly to the advantage of the cottager, so that it is a matter of great surprise that much more is not obtained. One swarm of bees, which may be

---

* The quantities are arranged, in these tables, in pounds and decimals, or tenths of a pound, and not in pounds and ounces. They may, however, be readily understood, for decimal 5 (or ·5) means half of ten, and therefore half of a pound, as each pound is divided into ten parts, and so on with the other quantities.

purchased for a few shillings, will produce others every year; and there is not the least difficulty in every cottager in the country paying a large part of his rent from this source alone—a source which scarcely gives him any trouble, and is tolerably sure. Our working classes have not realised the advantages which they might gain from it, as well as from the keeping of fowls, to which we shall hereafter refer, and by so doing they lose several pounds yearly. Let every householder keep hives, and increase the number with every swarm of bees.

Honey was formerly much used in this country in the production of a kind of wine called mead, as well as to sweeten food, before sugar had been introduced; but now it is more profitably sold as a luxury to those who wish to eat sweets with their bread and butter, at tea or breakfast. It is a very good kind of sugar, but too luscious to be eaten in large quantities without disordering the stomach.

It is always desirable to bear in mind that it may have poisonous qualities if flowers of a certain kind abound in the neighbourhood; and should it produce unusual effects, as sickness and giddiness, when taken in moderate quantities, it should be discontinued. The best honey is obtained where there is a great variety of flowers, including, particularly, clover and heather.

FAT.

Fat and oil are similar substances, but the first remains solid, except in very hot, and the latter, fluid, except in very cold weather.

The fat of flesh is enclosed in little bags or cells (Figs. 1 to 3), so that it is usual to cut lumps into small pieces, to allow the fat to run out more readily when it is made hot. The hardest is called suet (Fig. 3). There is also fat in many vegetables, and particularly in nuts, and this

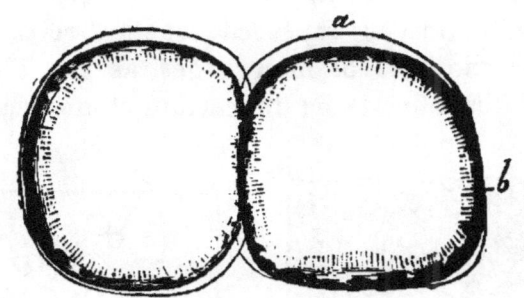

Fig. 1.
FAT CELLS IN MAN.
Showing the cell or bag *a*, and the contained semi-solid fat *b*.

also is found in little bags or cells. A very large quantity is made from the nut of the palm-tree, the cocoa-nut and the

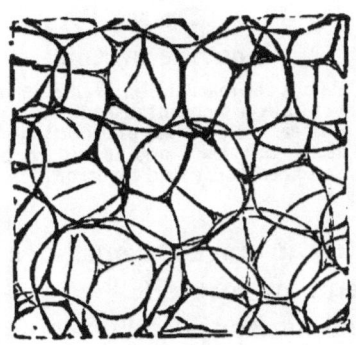 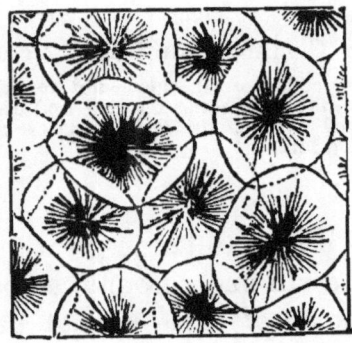

Fig. 2.
FAT CELLS.
These represent a number of cells or bags filled with fat.

Fig. 3.
FAT CELLS.
Showing solid fat in a crystalline form in the cells.

butter-nut, and much is now made from decayed vegetables in peat (Fig. 4).

Oil is found in nearly every part of an animal, but particularly about the skin and feet, as whale oil, seal oil, and neat's-foot oil; in the liver of fishes, as cod-liver oil; in the milk of animals, as the butter in cow's milk (Fig. 5); in the seeds of all plants, as linseed, rapeseed, mustard-seed, and cotton-seed oil; in the fruit of many trees, as the olive oil from the berry of the olive-tree; in certain stones called shales;

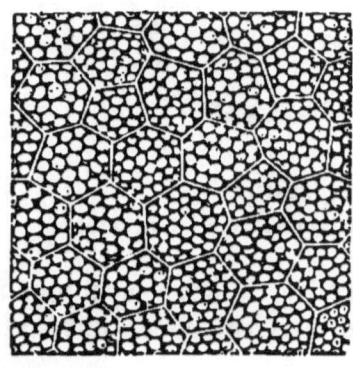

Fig. 4.

FAT CELLS OF THE COCOA NUT.

These cells are six-sided—not round, as in the preceding figures—and are filled with many small masses of solid fat.

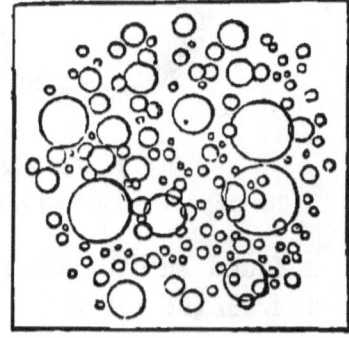

Fig. 5.

GLOBULES OF OIL.

This cut represents the cream in milk before it is separated and made into butter. It consists of globules of all sizes, and each one is said to have an exceedingly fine covering.

and it is collected in great quantities in cracks or openings in the earth underground, as petroleum or rock oil.

Some of these cannot be used as food in this country because they are not of an agreeable flavour; but as the taste of people varies, and particularly in different parts of the world, the inhabitants of cold countries eat whale oil and even tallow, whilst in this country we like the fresh fat of the flesh of animals, butter from milk, and the dripping from roasted meat, and in hot countries they prefer oil to fat.

Some people cannot eat every kind of fat of animals, but

FAT.

only one, as butter or the fat of bacon, whilst others can eat every kind in ordinary use. Some eat very little fat, and even greatly dislike fats generally, whilst others are very fond of them; but probably nobody exists who does not eat some quantity. It is not a sign of good health to refuse to eat fat generally, for fat is necessary, and we should eat probably from one to three ounces of it daily.

But few persons know how much fat they eat in the different foods which do not appear to contain fat, as well as in flesh, and the following table may be useful to them.

TABLE No. 2.

Table showing the number of pounds of fat in 100 pounds of the following foods :—

	lbs.
Potatoes, Carrots	0·2
Parsnips	0·5
Butter Milk and Rice	0·7
Bread	1·6
Skim Milk	1·8
Wheat Flour and Rye Meal	2·0
Peas	2·1
Barley Meal	2·4
White Fish	2·9
Lean Beef	3·6
Parsley	3·8
Ox Liver	4·1
Lean Mutton	4·9
Salmon	5·5
Oatmeal	5·6
Skim Milk Cheese	6·3
Indian Meal	8·1
Egg	10·5
Eels	13·8
Veal	15·3
Tripe	16·4
Cream	26·7
Fat Beef	29·3
Yolk of Egg	30·7
Cheddar Cheese and Fat Mutton	31·1
Fat Pork	48·9

	lbs.
Pickled Bacon	66·8
Dried Bacon	73·3
Butter, Dripping, and similar fats	83·0

Children who dislike fat cause much anxiety to parents, for they are almost always thin, and if not diseased, are not healthy. If care be not taken, they fall into a scrofulous condition, in which diseased joints, enlarged glands, sore eyes, and even consumption occur, and every effort should be made to overcome this dislike.

If attention be given to the foregoing remarks, there need be no anxiety about the possibility of increasing the quantity consumed, whilst with neglect, the dislike will probably increase until disease is produced. The chief period of growth —viz., from seven to sixteen years of age—is the most important in this respect, for a store of fat in the body is then essential.

Those who are inclined to be fat usually like fat in food, and then it may be desirable to limit its use. But to this we shall again refer.

Some who cannot eat it when hot like it when cold, and all should select that kind which they prefer. Those living in Russia and Lapland devour very large quantities, as seven pounds daily, and eat it even raw, whilst those dwelling in hot countries use very little. It produces more heat than any other kind of food.

STARCH.

Every one knows starch as it is used in stiffening linen, but does not know that he eats a great quantity of it every day. It is found largely in all kinds of grain, as wheat and rice, whilst sago, arrowroot, and tapioca are made almost entirely of it and water. It is in bags or cells, which can be seen only by the microscope, and as the cells of each kind differ from every other in size and form, or in their markings, one can say

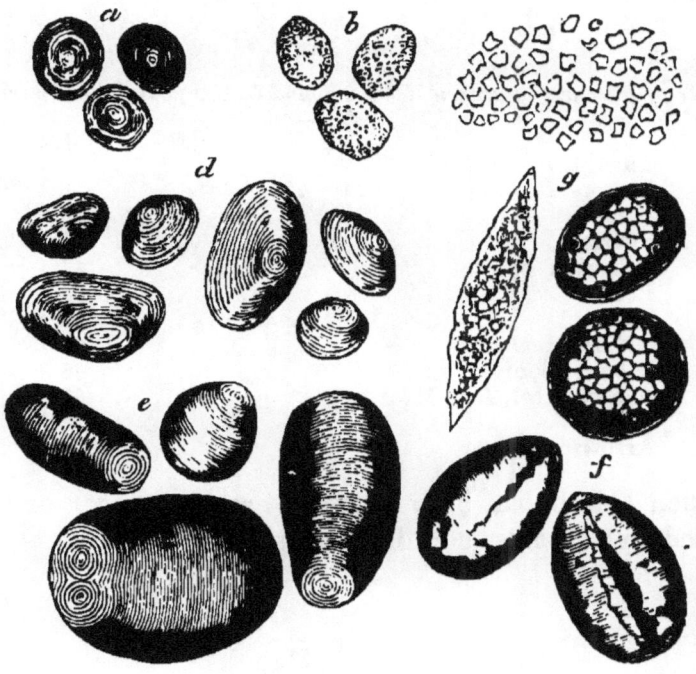

Fig. 6.
STARCH CELLS (*magnified*).

a, wheat; *b*, sago; *c*, rice; *d*, potato; *e*, tous les mois; *f*, Cell wall ruptured by dry heat; *g*, cells of the rhubarb containing starch granules.

whether a starch cell is from rice, or wheat, &c., as in Fig. 6. When, however, the starch has been removed from the bag, it is no longer possible to say from what plant it was obtained, for it is the same from every kind of food.

It is not at all difficult to separate the starch from other substances associated with it, for if fine flour be well washed in water the starch falls to the bottom, and may be removed and dried. It is thus that starch is made in this country, and in preparing arrowroot and sago in other countries.

This is the greatest proportion of our solid food from vegetables, and we eat from four ounces to one pound of it daily.

TABLE No. 3.

Number of pounds of starch which are found in 100 pounds of the following foods:—

	lbs.
Turnips	5·1
Carrots	8·4
Parsnips	9·6
Potatoes	18·8
Wheaten Bread	47·4
Peas	55·4
Oatmeal	58·4
Indian Meal	64·7
Wheat Flour	66·3
Barley Meal, Rye Meal	69·4
Rice	79·1
Arrowroot	82·0

When starch has been eaten it becomes sugar or fat in the body, or it may be entirely consumed.

FLOUR.

Flour is made by grinding seeds, as wheat, when it is commonly called flour; and oats, barley, and rye, when it is called meal.

Wheat flour is preferred to every other for its flavour, and it is practically the most nourishing of all grains.

Oatmeal is a very strong and good food, but is not much eaten in this country. This is not owing to want of nutritive value, but to its higher price as compared with wheat-flour, and to a rougher flavour, so that children, as they grow up, prefer wheat flour to it. It is, however, still eaten as a daily food in the colder parts of our country, as in the Highlands or Islands of Scotland, and the Peak of Derbyshire, as well as in certain very poor districts, as parts of South Wales and Ireland; but it will never again come into general use.

Barley meal is eaten in some parts of Wales either alone or with wheat flour, but is a much poorer food than wheat flour.

Rye meal is eaten in some parts of Yorkshire and the northern counties of England, and is almost always mixed with wheat flour, but in many parts of Europe the poorer people eat it alone.

Every seed has a skin and kernel, and when it is ground the flour is a mixture of both; but nearly all the skin can be removed by sifting, and in proportion as it is removed the flour becomes whiter. Fine flour means that from which all or nearly all the skin has been sifted out; seconds, or household, that which has more of the skin; thirds have more still, and batch, or brown flour, has all, or nearly all, the skin left in it. The skin is divided into several parts, which are sold as bran or sharps, for the food of animals, but there are always small pieces of the kernel with them. The bran, when it is eaten by man, is liable to purge, and is better left out of the flour.

There is none of these foods so good and cheap as good seconds wheat flour, except where wheat does not grow, and is costly to buy.

Flour consists chiefly of starch, with some sugar and gluten, or bird-lime, besides various salts.

The flour of wheat and oatmeal is made into puddings, and that of wheat, rye, and barley into bread. When flour is boiled in water the starch cells (Fig. 6) burst and the starch escapes and thickens the water; but oatmeal requires to be boiled longer than wheat flour because its starch cells do not burst so readily. Both kinds, however, should be well boiled. When yeast is added (Fig. 7) the flour ferments and becomes light and spongy. Yeast dumplings are made with this dough boiled in water, but they should not be boiled too long, or they will become less light and not so digestible.

Flour mixed with fat, baking-powder, or egg-powder, is rolled into thin layers and made into piecrust, but it is not easily digested if too much fat be used. When mixed with suet chopped into small portions it may be boiled or baked as suet pudding, or made into the crust of boiled meat or fruit pies, or it may be rolled into layers and wrapped up with treacle or preserves in roley-poley puddings. The pieces of suet should not be too large, nor so small that when cooked they cannot be seen. Pastry made with butter or fat may be eaten when both hot and cold, but when with suet it should be eaten hot.

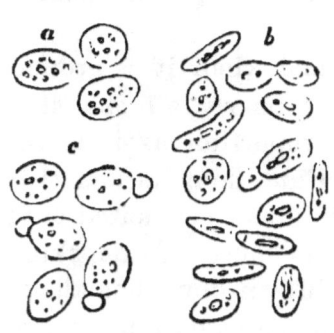

Fig. 7.
YEAST CELLS.

They are little bags which are filled with granules, and multiply by division as in c, each part becoming a separate and perfect cell.

Wheaten flour is often adulterated with cheaper foods, as rice flour, or with stronger foods, as pea-meal, or with useless substances, as Paris plaster; but more commonly an inferior kind of wheat flour, as that of wheat which has sprouted, is added to it, when it is said to be unsound.

DRIED PEAS, BEANS, AND LENTILS.

These are said to be the strongest of all vegetable foods, because they contain the greatest proportion of that substance (nitrogen) which repairs the body, and in this respect they are very like skimmed milk cheese in animal foods. They are, no doubt, very nourishing and sustaining, but the flavour is somewhat harsh and strong; and children, particularly, do not like them so well as potatoes or bread. Those who are very poor should use them in proportion to their cheapness on account of the nourishment which they give.

A few observations should be borne in mind when they are cooked and eaten.

1. The shells should be taken out, since they are not digestible, and will be very likely to disturb the bowels.

2. They should be well boiled, but not to a perfect pulp, lest when they are strained their form cannot be distinguished.

3. They should be cooked or eaten with fat or bacon liquor, since they are very deficient in fat.

4. They should be properly seasoned, and if onions, turnips, or similar fresh vegetables, be cooked and eaten with them, their flavour will be disguised.

5. Do not eat food made of peas too frequently.

Pease-pudding is a very good food when eaten with fat. Broad beans are not eaten when they are dried, but a small kind like the kidney-bean (haricots) are much used in other countries, and have a more agreeable flavour than peas.

When fresh vegetables are scarce, as in the winter, this kind of food is more generally eaten. The German soldiers, in their late war with France, were fed chiefly on sausages made of peas, bacon, and dried meat.

Lentils, or pulse, are much eaten in other countries, and are equally good food with peas and beans.

BREAD.

Bread is generally made into loaves or cakes of some inches in thickness, as in ordinary wheaten, rye, and barley bread;

but oatmeal can be made into thin cakes only. It is prepared by adding water, yeast (Fig. 7), and salt, to flour, and when the dough begins to rise it is put into the oven and baked. Sometimes baking-powder is used instead of yeast, and makes the bread light; but it is not so good. The yeast may be either fluid, as brewer's barm; or almost dry, as German yeast; and both, if good, cause fermentation equally well.

When bread is to be made, the flour is thrown into a vessel, and well mixed with a proper quantity of salt. A space is then made in the middle, in which warm water and yeast are placed, and the flour is gradually mixed with them until the whole is made into dough, when it is well kneaded, and placed before the fire until it begins to rise. It should be lightly covered, and not made too hot, and it should not be allowed to rise too much. When it is ready, it is taken out and quickly made into cakes, or placed in tins, and is ready for the oven.

The heat of the oven should not be too little, or the bread will be close and sodden, nor too great, or it will be too much dried, or even burnt; and when the cake will ring on being struck with the knuckles, it is sufficiently baked.

About two ounces of salt and three pints of water are required for each fourteen pounds of flour.

The water makes the starch cells swell, and perhaps burst. The yeast, or baking-powder, mixes air or a gas with the dough, and by separating it, makes the dough light and spongy, but in doing so, the yeast (not the baking-powder) wastes some of the flour. The heat in the baking helps to burst the starch cells, and drives off so much of the water as to make the bread agreeably dry. If too much water is left the bread is too moist, and is disagreeable; and if too little, the bread is dry and hard, and has lost much of its flavour, and some of its nutriment. The more water is left the heavier is the bread made from a stone of flour, and the less water the lighter is the weight of bread. 14 lb. of flour should make 19 lb. to 20 lb. of bread. When bread is bought it should not be too moist, as it becomes drier by keeping. It should be a day old, but when home made, it may be kept several days with advantage.

When it is baked or bought it should be kept in a dry place where the air is fresh and good, for it absorbs air and might become unwholesome.

Bread made from good seconds wheat flour gives the most nourishment for the money expended, but in many places rye-flour or barley-meal costs much less and is added to it. There is less nourishment in such a mixture than in wheat flour alone, but it is often very agreeable as a change of food, and rye keeps the bread moist.

Brown bread, rye bread, or barley bread do not agree so well with children as white wheaten bread.

Bread is very frequently adulterated with alum to make it take up more water, and by green copperas to make it whiter. The alum is easily shown by dipping a slice of bread into a weak watery solution of logwood, when it becomes of a purplish tint. The logwood infusion is made by putting a few pieces of logwood into boiling water, and allowing it to stand for three or four hours by the fire. The colour of the infusion must not be deep.

Oatmeal is not made into loaves because the starch cells do not easily burst, and it is not possible to cook it well in a thick mass; but it is made into thin cakes from a quarter to half an inch thick. The oatmeal is mixed with water, yeast, and salt, as in making loaves of bread, and the dough is then spread out into a thin layer and baked on a hot iron plate or stone. If the water has not well soaked into the meal the cakes will be hard, gritty, and dry, and if too much water be left the cakes will become sour. When properly made they may be kept good for months.

When neither yeast nor baking-powder is added to the flour or meal the bread or cake is unloavened, and must be made thin and baked so as to be crisp. This kind of cake is eaten by the Jews at the period of the Passover.

Pearl barley and Scotch barley are creed by being soaked in water, and are then boiled in milk or made into puddings.

Wheat which has been steeped in water and then boiled in milk, and spiced, is called frumenty or frumity, and was in use a thousand years ago.

It may interest the young reader to know how it was made in 1350, and to read the English words of that time—

"Nym (*take*) clene, wete and bray (*bruise*) it in a morter wel, that the holys (*hulls or shells*) gon al of, and seethe (*soak or simmer*) yt til it breste (*burst*), and nym yt up and lat it kele (*cool*), and nym fayre fresh broth and swete mylk of almandys (*almonds*) or swete mylk of kyne (*cows*), and temper (*mix*) it al, and nym the yolkys of eyryn (*eggs*); boyle it a lityl, and set yt ad on and messe yt forthe wyth fat venyson and fresh moton (*mutton*)."

They are very good and agreeable foods.

RICE, SAGO, ARROWROOT, AND TAPIOCA.

These foods are not grown in England, and are therefore brought here in a dry state, and are almost exclusively used in making puddings.

Rice (Fig. 6) grows and is thrashed and winnowed as we grow and prepare wheat, and is eaten, instead of wheat, by hundreds of millions of people in hot countries, where wheat is

RICE, SAGO, ARROWROOT, AND TAPIOCA.

but little known. It is not so good a food as wheat, because it has very little gluten (or bird-lime), and is almost entirely composed of starch. When it is ground the flour does not stick together, so that it could not be made into loaves, but as it is sometimes cheaper than wheat and is whiter, it is added to wheaten flour to adulterate it. This is wrong, because it is not so good a food as ordinary flour, and by making the flour whiter the purchaser is led to think that it is finer and better than ordinary flour. When it is eaten instead of bread it is not ground, but the whole rice is boiled in water until it is soft, and it is then eaten alone, or with meat or fat. It should not be so much boiled as to fall to pieces, or much of the starch will be lost in the water and thrown away, whilst the rice would not be so agreeable to the taste; but it should be cooked enough to be softened throughout, and not to taste hard or gritty.

Different kinds of rice vary more in this respect than in the nutriment which they give, so that some, as the Carolina rice, swell, thicken, and improve in flavour, whilst others, as the Patna rice, swell but little, and are apt to have a dry taste.

When rice is made into puddings with milk, sugar, and spice, it is more agreeable and nourishing. It should be well cooked, but if too much so, there will be waste of the milk, and the sugar will not be so sweet.

Rice is not so cheap as flour when bought retail, having regard to its power to nourish, and should not be largely used by the poor.

Sago, arrowroot, and tapioca (Fig. 6) are not grains like rice or wheat. Sago is obtained by beating the stem of a palm-tree, and arrowroot by beating the root of a tree, and in both cases the matter thrashed out is washed and dried.

The preparation of arrowroot is interesting, inasmuch as

the juice of the root is so highly injurious to life that the Indians dip arrows into it in order to make them poisonous. The following description of the process is quoted from my work on botany:—

"In a dense forest of Guiana the Indian chief has stretched his sleeping-mat between two high stems of the magnolia. He rests indolently smoking beneath the shade of the broad-leaved banana, gazing at the doings of his family around. His wife pounds the gathered mandioc-roots with a wooden club, in the hollow-trunk of a tree, and wraps the thick pulp in a compact net made from the tough leaves of the great lily plants. The long bundle is hung upon a stick which rests on two forks, and a heavy stone is fastened to the bottom, the weight of which causes the juice to be pressed out. This runs into a shell of the calabash gourd placed beneath. Close by, squats a little boy, and dips his father's arrows in the deadly milk, while the wife lights a fire to dry the pressed roots, and by heat to drive off more completely the volatile poisonous matter.

"Next, it is powdered between two stones, and the casava meal is ready. Meanwhile the boy has completed his evil task; the sap after standing some considerable time has deposited a delicate white starch, from which the poisonous fluid is poured off. The meal is then well washed with water, and is the fine tapioca, resembling in every respect arrowroot."

When you next eat a tapioca or arrowroot pudding remember how closely life and death are associated.

These substances contain scarcely anything but starch and water, and are not therefore so nourishing as rice, much less as wheat. They are not made into bread or pastry, but only into puddings, either with water alone, when they are very poor food, or with milk and spice, when they are a very agreeable food, particularly for children. They should be well cooked. Arrowroot is very dear, and not at all equal to flour in nutriment, yet it is very foolishly given in the belief that it is very nourishing, and thereby many young children are ill-fed. It is much used by the sick when prepared with milk or wine.

FRESH VEGETABLES.

Fresh vegetables—as potatoes, cabbage, greens, carrots, parsnips, and turnips—are very necessary foods, and by their juices prevent disease. Turnip-tops, nettles, spinach, and a great variety of green herbs, are valuable for the latter purpose when fresh and young.

None is so useful as the potato, because it is the most nutritious; but even potato, when eaten alone, is a poor food, and not equal to rice, much less to flour. It is cheap when grown by the cottager by his own labour and in his own garden; but when bought, it is much dearer than bread, having regard to its nutriment only. Hence, whilst it is a necessary food, it is not always cheap, and should not be purchased in too large a quantity. Half a pound a day is probably enough for each person, and when green vegetables are plentiful, bread may be eaten instead of it. When eaten in large quantities, as in Wales or Ireland, butter-milk or milk should be eaten with it. The allowance at a farm-house in Ireland is ten and a half pounds of potato and three and a half pints of butter-milk daily.

There are many kinds of potato, but two are particularly distinguished in cooking, viz., mealy and waxy, and persons differ much in their taste respecting them. The mealy are perhaps generally preferred, but as they boil down and break to pieces readily, they are less economical than the waxy.

When cooked by boiling, they may be either soft throughout, as is preferred in England, or a little hard in the centre, as in Ireland. When baked alone, they should be well cooked in their skins, so as to break down into a powder throughout, but when peeled and baked in fat, they remain whole. If cooked in their skins, there is less waste than when peeled first, but the waxy do not look so well after peeling as the mealy.

A good kind of potato is heavy in proportion to its size, which shows that it is starchy rather than waxy. This is readily ascertained by lifting it in the hand as you would judge of an orange.

Potatoes should be eaten with fat and salt, meat or milk.

The increase in the price of potatoes of late years has been due to the "potato disease," by which the crop has been greatly reduced in quantity, and the gathered potatoes have subsequently become unsound. This was the immediate cause of the famine, attended with great loss of life, in Ireland, in 1845, since the people provided no other food in sufficient quantity for their use, and when it failed they were absolutely destitute. That great calamity, however, has borne good fruit, by leading the inhabitants of Ireland, Scotland, and Wales to rely less upon that article of diet, and to provide themselves with Indian corn, oatmeal, or other food of higher nutritive character.

The disease still remains in a limited degree, and its possible occurrence is a subject of anxiety every year. Its nature has not been satisfactorily determined, but it is first seen in the removal of the starch from the cells of the potato, and then by the presence of a fungus. Some affirm that the fungus is the cause, and others the effect, of the disease.

These changes are well shown in Figs. 8, 9, and 10.

It is sometimes possible to separate the part of a potato

which is diseased from that which is sound, and to use the latter for food, but not infrequently the disease extends farther than can be seen by the naked eye, and it has been found more economical and healthful to give the whole potato to the pigs.

All green vegetables require to be well boiled, and the green colour should be preserved by adding a little soda to the water. The fresher they are, the better the flavour and colour. Cabbage is the cheapest of all garden green

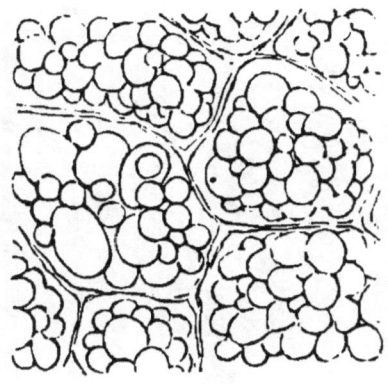

Fig. 8.
SECTION OF HEALTHY POTATO.
Starch cells of different sizes are seen enclosed in the cells of the potato.

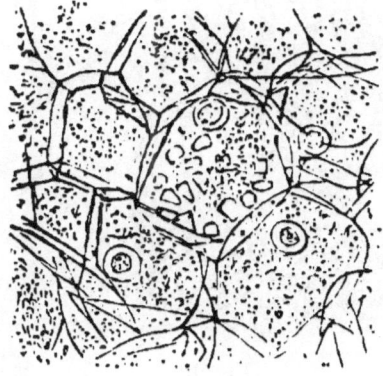

Fig. 9.
SECTION OF DISEASED POTATO.
Nearly all the starch cells have been destroyed, and the potato cells are empty. Such a potato is valueless.

vegetables, and should be grown freely; and whether fried or boiled, it should be well cooked. Turnip-tops are the cheapest and best of field green vegetables, and should be eaten freely.

Carrots and parsnips are better food than turnips, as they contain more sugar, fat, and starch, but they are dearer. White turnip is preferred to the Swede, because of its more agreeable flavour, but it is not so nourishing. All are used more to flavour food than as food; but every kind of fresh vegetable that is good for food, should be eaten as freely as possible.

There is much needless waste in the use of vegetables, for by peeling and cutting, the potato is often reduced to half its former size, and much is lost in throwing away the outside leaves of cabbage, lettuce, and celery. The parts which are thus cut away may not be so tender and agreeable as that which remains, but they are good food, and if not

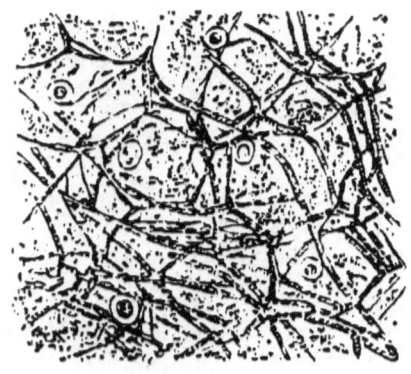

Fig. 10.
SECTION OF DISEASED POTATO.

The cells of the potato are occupied by a fungus, as shown by the thick lines which traverse the cut. Such a potato might give rise to disease.

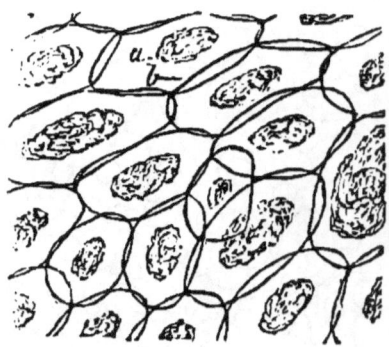

Fig. 11.
STRAWBERRY CELLS.

The cells lie loosely amongst each other, and are not pressed together as in Fig. 4. Each contains a small quantity of solid matter, and is then filled with juice.

given to the pigs are really wasted. These foods are very costly in towns, and servants should be careful in preparing them.

Fruits of every kind which are used as food, should be eaten in their season, for their juices are very agreeable and useful, although not very nutritious. Such are apples, pears, gooseberries, strawberries, and all our garden fruits (Fig. 11). All may be eaten when either raw or cooked, but some—as apples and pears—are more easily digested when cooked, and should not be eaten raw in large quantities. In the middle of summer, too much fresh fruit may cause diarrhœa or purging, and do harm, but it is less likely to do so if cooked and eaten with sugar; and if it should occur, a tea-spoonful of brandy, or a little strong wine, will generally arrest it at first. When cooking them in pies or puddings, it is cheaper to add the sugar after cooking, as the heat lessens the sweetness of the sugar. So also when making preserves, the sugar should not be boiled too long, or it will be injured.

The quantity of sugar which is found in different kinds of fruits differs much, and it also varies with the degree of ripeness.

TABLE No. 4.

Table showing the number of pounds of sugar in 100 lbs. of the following fruits:—

	lbs.
Strawberries, Wild	4·5
,, Cultivated	7·5
Raspberries, Wild	3·5
,, Cultivated	4·7
Apples, English rennett	6·8
,, White dessert	7·5
,, English golden pippin	10·6
Pears, sweet red	7·9
Cherries, sour	8·7
,, sweet black	10·7
,, sweet light red	13·1
Blackberries	4·4
Bilberries	5·7
Mulberries	9·2
Grapes	from 10 to 20

Dried fruits, as currants, raisins, dates, figs, and prunes, are very pleasant, but are used rather to give an agreeable flavour to flour than to nourish the body, and are dear foods. Dates contain more than half their weight of sugar.

BUTCHERS' MEAT.

The lean meat of every animal which is sold by the butcher is nearly equally nourishing, but differs in the quickness with which it is digested. Thus, pork and veal are said to be indigestible, whilst mutton is more quickly digested than beef; so that, as a general rule, people prefer mutton and beef. This is, however, due to the difficulty of chewing pork and veal, and as people do not take sufficient care, they swallow it in large pieces. All kinds of meat—but particularly these—should be chewed slowly, and be completely masticated before they are swallowed. It is also better to cut it into very small pieces before putting it into the mouth. Some who eat large pieces at once, and do not chew it until it is quite broken up, swallow large lumps which stop in the throat and choke them, so that they die. Whenever any one does this, somebody should push his finger down the throat, and try to pull out the piece, but this should be done at once, as he will die in three to five minutes if he cannot breathe. It is of no use to wait for a doctor to come.

Pork and veal are, however, much liked for their flavour, and they should be particularly well cooked, so as to be more easily chewed and digested. Pork is more commonly diseased than any other kind of meat, and on that account also should be well cooked. Any meat which is softer, more watery, much darker or much lighter

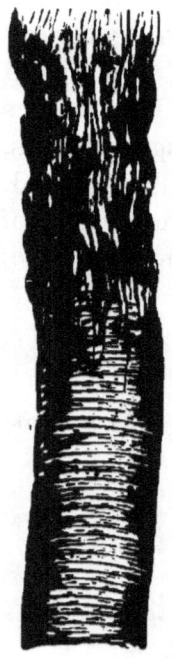

Fig. 12.
STRIATED MUSCULAR FIBRE.

Flesh consists of bundles of fibres, as shown in Fig. 12, which have generally a number of cross lines, called *striæ*, A, and are made up of hundreds of smaller fibres, or *fibrillæ*, as shown at B in colour than ordinary meat, or which has small bladders in it, or anything unusual in the appearance or smell, is probably diseased, and should not be eaten.

Dr. Letheby gives the following advice in the selection of meat:—

"Good meat has the following characters:—

1. "It is neither of a pale pink colour nor of a deep purple tint, for the former is a sign of disease and the latter indicates that the animal has not been slaughtered, but has died with the blood in it, or has suffered from acute fever.

2. "It has a marbled appearance from the ramifications of little veins of fat among the muscles.

3. "It should be firm and elastic to the touch, and should scarcely moisten the fingers — bad meat being wet and sodden and flabby, with the fat looking like jelly or wet parchment.

4. "It should have little or no odour, and the odour should not be disagreeable, for diseased meat has a sickly cadaverous smell, and sometimes a smell of physic. This is very discoverable when the meat is chopped up and drenched with warm water.

5. "It should not shrink much in cooking.

6. "It should not run to water or become very wet on standing for a day or so, but should, on the contrary, dry upon the surface.

7. "When dried at a temperature of 212 degrees (boiling point) or thereabout, it should not lose more than 70 to 74 per cent. of its weight, whereas bad meat will often lose as much as 80 per cent."

Pork, veal, and mutton pies and sausages, are sometimes made of diseased meat, and all such should be regarded with suspicion, unless the maker be well known to be honest and respectable.

When meat is cooked it loses weight, but if it be roasted or baked, and not overdone, it loses water chiefly, and still retains nearly all the nourishment; so that ¾ lb. of cooked, with the dripping, will be as nourishing as 1 lb. of fresh meat. When it is boiled, the juice goes into the broth, and nothing is lost if both the meat and broth be eaten. The broth should never be thrown away, but eaten with fresh vegetables and rice, or pearl barley.

When meat is over-roasted it is wasted, and what is left will be less nourishing. When it is underdone it is not so agreeable to the taste or so easy to chew. The outside will always be more done than the inside, and the inside may be reddish in colour and yet sufficiently cooked. When cooking meat, too much of the juices should not be drawn out, and if the outside be quickly cooked or hardened, it prevents their escape. Therefore, when meat is roasted it should be put near the fire for a few minutes to harden the outside, and then drawn a little back for the rest of the cooking; and, when boiled, it should be put into boiling water for perhaps five minutes, and then drawn from the fire a little so as to prevent it boiling again. When meat is kept boiling it is made hard throughout, and is neither so agreeable nor so tender and nourishing. It can be cooked perfectly well without being boiled, and when it is simmered only.

If you want to make very good broth or soup, do not boil the meat at all, but let it only simmer; but the better the broth the less nourishing is the meat. So, if you want the meat to be as nourishing as possible, put it, as just stated, into boiling water, and then draw the pot back.

The dripping from roasted and baked meat, and the fat on broth, should be carefully saved and eaten, as they are very useful foods.

Salting always injures meat, because it draws out the juices, which, being too salt, cannot be eaten. Moreover, too much salt is not good for health. When, however, meat is properly salted, it is very agreeable, although not so nourishing. Unless the flavour of salted meat is required, or, as in hot weather, the meat will not keep, it should not be salted, but eaten fresh; yet the use of a little salt rubbed once on a piece of pork will not do any great harm, whilst it will improve the flavour. Salted meat is always a dear and wasteful food as compared with fresh meat; yet in some parts of the country, where the poorer classes eat pork only, it is necessary to put it into pickle, and thus they keep it good through many months. A good pickle is made by adding three pounds of salt and a quarter of a pound of saltpetre to a gallon of water, and may be kept and used for a long time.

But although all meat is nearly equally good as food, the different joints vary in flavour and tenderness, and some are preferred to others. Thus, the back loin of beef and leg of mutton are preferred to all other joints, and are therefore the dearest; but cheaper joints, which have less flavour and are coarser, may be equally nourishing. A poor person should therefore buy the cheaper joints, and make them tender by good cooking, and agreeable by flavouring them properly.

In selecting joints there are two other conditions to bear in mind, viz., the proportion of fat and bone. Fat is very useful, but is quite different in its nourishing powers from lean flesh, and a very fat joint, as the neck of mutton, is not so economical at half the price as the leg without much fat. Yet as persons differ much in eating fat, those who like it may buy the fat parts and others should buy the lean. A fat leg of mutton is not so economical as a lean one, if both are well fed, and generally joints with much fat are not cheap.

As to bone, every one knows that it is not so valuable as meat, and that a joint with much bone sells for less than one with little. Thus the aitch-bone has some of the best-flavoured meat, but it has also a large bone, and is therefore sold at a lower price; whilst the leg of mutton has very little bone in proportion to the meat, and is sold at a high price. That joint is the most economical which has the least bone and fat in moderate quantity. The thin ribs of beef may have little bone, but they have much fat, whilst the round and the thick flank may be entirely without bone.

But bones are valuable as food when properly cooked.

It is better to keep the meat for a short time than to eat it when quite fresh, and if it becomes drier it loses only water and is none the worse. It should not, however, be kept until it smells disagreeably. Meat which has been kept a little too long should be roasted rather than boiled.

UNCOOKED MEAT.

It is not a frequent habit in this country to eat uncooked meat or flesh, but sometimes butchers' boys and others eat thin slices of raw meat. In other countries, however, it is not uncommon to eat ham, salted legs of mutton, and dried and smoked beef raw, besides eating sausages which are made of all sorts of meat, either raw or very insufficiently cooked; and the people say that uncooked meat gives more strength than when it is cooked.

No doubt uncooked meat may be digested by the stomach, and some nourishment may be lost in cooking it; but there are sometimes little worms and other creatures in meat which are changed into other kinds of worms in our bodies if they are eaten alive, and cause the most frightful diseases. It is therefore far better to lose a little nourishment by cooking the meat than to have such terrible results from eating it raw; and all meat, whether fresh, salted, or dried, should be cooked before it is eaten.

Many people in Germany and elsewhere have had 50,000 worms in one inch of their flesh after having eaten of diseased and uncooked meat. These minute thread-like creatures have penetrated everywhere, even into the eyes, and caused death.

OFFAL.

What is called the offal of meat is usually good food. Such are the head, heart, lungs, liver, and other parts called the fry, and the feet, and they are always cheaper than the same weight of meat. Sometimes the liver and lungs are diseased, and they should be carefully examined and all bladders and glands cut out. They should also be well cooked. The head makes excellent soup or broth. The heart is very economical, but it is not so full of flavour or so easily chewed as other kinds of meat. The feet are very gelatinous and are agreeable and useful food. Tripe is quickly digested and not very nourishing, but it is easily prepared and is agreeable.

Blood is not so much used in the country as in towns, but when made into black-puddings, with barley or groats, fat and seasoning, is very good and agreeable food. Where pigs are killed the blood should be saved and eaten in this way, and the pudding-skins are easily obtained from the bowels when well washed. It has long been the practice of families in Scotland to make a quantity of black puddings at Michaelmas for use during the winter, and to hang them in strings to the roof until required for use. Two or three pounds of blood are nearly equal to one pound of meat.

Tripe and cowheel are favourite foods in towns, and may be readily prepared, but should be well cleaned and boiled. It is very doubtful whether much more food for man could not be obtained from these sources, for at present a much greater proportion goes to the dog kennel and to the glue boiler than is desirable, and but few housewives in villages either properly value them or will take the trouble to obtain and clean them. It is quite true that being so quickly digested they are not fitted for a principal meal, but they are at least valuable at supper, and also at dinner to those poor who cannot obtain flesh. The oil which is obtained from the cowheel has too strong a flavour to be used as food, but is valuable for other purposes.

It is very desirable that the true value of this large class of foods should be better understood by the poor, in order that much food which is now lost to man may be retained.. The prejudices of many are giving way since more persons will now eat blood than formerly, and the nutritive value of these and every other kinds of food is better known.

GELATIN AND ISINGLASS.

Gelatin is made from many substances which do not appear to be food, as the skin, bones, hoofs, and horns of animals, and is therefore so much food saved from waste. It is prepared by boiling them to separate it from other matters, after which it is clarified or decolorised, dried and cut into strings. When again dissolved in warm water it swells and acquires more than its original bulk. It is nearly tasteless, and therefore requires lemon juice, wine, or other condiments to be added. It is animal food of valuable qualities, but not so good as meat, and is probably inferior to both fish and egg. It is never relied upon to furnish a meal.

Isinglass is a purer gelatin, obtained from the sound or air-bladder of a fish called the sturgeon, which is caught in the Russian seas, and from its comparative rarity is much dearer than ordinary gelatin. It is also preferred as to its taste, and it will make a firmer jelly than the same weight of ordinary gelatin, but these advantages are not at all equal to the greatly increased cost.

BACON.

Bacon is cheap in this country only when it is made from a pig reared by the eater from waste food, and attended to in his spare time, for it is now sold at a high price, and consists chiefly of fat, which is less nourishing than flesh. It is, however, very agreeable, and supplies the place of butter or other fat, but it is not sufficient alone to maintain strength of body. In some counties nearly every cottager has a garden and pig, and thus having food in the house when he may not have money wherewith to buy fresh meat, finds it very useful.

It is desirable that every poor person in the country who can keep a pig from his own garden, without annoying or injuring his neighbour, should do so, and thus save and lay by money or money's worth.

Bacon may be either fried or boiled. If the former, the fluid fat or dripping should be eaten at the same time, and if the latter, cabbage or beans should be boiled with it, and thus save the fat and flavour which have been boiled out of the bacon. Bacon-liquor, however, is not rich enough alone to make broth, but is good when meat is boiled in it. It should not be thrown away, for if not eaten the fat may be skimmed off and used in cooking.

The lean of bacon is generally hard and tough, and is not easily chewed. It must be cut into thin rashers if fried, but when well and gently boiled in a lump, it becomes tender, and has a delicious flavour. Shoulder of bacon, or ham, requires very gentle and careful cooking to make it as tender and agreeable as possible. Bacon is, however, generally preferred for its fat, and is more or less agreeable as the pig was well or ill-fed, and the bacon well or carelessly salted and dried.

There are many agricultural counties where bacon is the only kind of meat which the labourer can obtain, and, then, in very small quantities, once or twice a week. Hence it is very much prized and liked by them, but it is not so nutritious as fresh meat in that quality which repairs the body, and is rarely if ever so cheap as the lower priced joints. Whilst, therefore, it is a very agreeable and useful food, every person should obtain fresh meat in preference, if their means will permit them to do so.

POULTRY AND GAME.

These are not so nourishing as butcher's meat, and, speaking generally, are much dearer. They are useful to the sick and the rich, yet a rabbit is often a cheap and agreeable dish to the poor. Most kinds of wild game are tougher than butcher's meat, and are made tender by being kept until they are a little disagreeable to the smell. Nearly all game should be roasted.

CHEESE.

Cheese is not a very digestible food, and should not be eaten in large quantities at a time; but a little makes other food digest. It is not a cheap food, although some kinds of skim-milk cheese may cost little, and whenever it is possible meat should be eaten instead of it. It is however an agreeable addition to bread. When it is made from new milk, it contains much fat, and is both cheese and butter, and is good food, but when from skim-milk there is little or no fat, and it is only cheese, and not a good food.

The use of cheese varies very much in different parts of the country, so that in South Wales and Wiltshire it is regarded as a necessary article of food, whilst in other counties the poor rarely eat it. This is partly due to habit, but chiefly to poverty, for where cheese is much eaten it is cheap and of inferior quality, and the people are too poor to buy meat. Hence a dinner of bread and cheese is exceedingly common, whilst one of meat and vegetables is extremely rare. The quantity of cheese eaten throughout the country is not diminishing, but almost everywhere cheese is eaten in small quantity at a time, as an addition to other foods, and rather as a luxury or relish than as a food. It is not desirable that it should be eaten alone, although it consists chiefly of that which repairs the body, and so far is the richest of all foods.

The best kinds made in this country are Stilton, Cheshire, double-Gloucester, and Cheddar, but others are nearly equally good. Some American cheese is very rich, but has a flavour which is not liked, whilst much of it is very strong and causes indigestion.

FISH.

Fish is a good food, but not equal to flesh in nourishing the body. Some kinds—as herrings—contain much fat, and are so far very useful, whilst at the same time they are very cheap. Others, as soles, have little fat, and are much dearer, or as whitings, which are often very cheap. Cod-fish is a good food and often cheap, but rarely so cheap as the lower priced joints of meat, in proportion to the nourishment afforded. The fat or oil is not so much in the flesh as in the liver, which is not much eaten.

Salmon in season is the most nourishing of all fish, and when it becomes plentiful and cheap, should be universally eaten. It has red blood, and is therefore more like butcher's meat, and contains a large quantity of oil, which is like the fat of flesh. When out of season, the fish is very thin and watery, and contains scarcely any oil.

Eels contain much oil, and are delicious but dear food.

On the whole, fish is not so much eaten in England, or so much cultivated in our rivers and ponds, as it ought to be; but as it soon perishes, the supply from the sea must be fitful, and its price vary much. It will, however, become plentiful and cheap.

Dried fish cannot be so cheap as fresh, but is nourishing, and a bloater is more agreeable than a fresh herring. It is, however, often cheaper than flesh, and more convenient to the poor both in town and country. When very highly salted it often causes indigestion.

The value of fish, in proportion to the nourishment which it affords, varies extremely with the kind and the abundance of the supply, and, therefore, with the locality and the weather, but it can never supplant meat.

Where fish is brought to the shore in large quantity it is

often possible to obtain it at a very low price, so that it may be the cheapest food obtainable; but if the inhabitants cannot purchase butcher's meat also, they will fall into disease. It is said that leprosy is found where fish is much and flesh very little eaten, and it is quite certain that indigestion, and a low state of health are there very common.

If fish can be obtained as a relish, or a change of food, it may be both agreeable and useful, but if it be the only kind of animal food, it is insufficient to maintain good health.

EGGS.

Eggs are very good food, and all persons who can should keep fowls. They are not equal to meat, although they are more like lean meat than fat in their action, and when the yolk is eaten with the white, there is oil which represents fat. Whenever they are cheap, they should be eaten freely, and they are equally nourishing whether poached, fried, or boiled. They differ, however, very much with the amount of cooking, so that a raw egg will be digested in $1\frac{1}{2}$ hours, whilst a hard-boiled or fried egg will require 3 or $3\frac{1}{2}$ hours. They should therefore not be made hard by cooking.

The eggs of all birds are of nearly the same value in nourishment in proportion to their size, but some, as those of the seagull, have a strong flavour, which is not liked. All large eggs should be used as food if they can be obtained fresh, but the eggs of small birds are wasted, and it is cruel to take them.

When eggs are fried, the pan should not be too hot, and there should first be a little butter, salt, and pepper put into it, and the egg carefully turned and made brown on both sides. The pan should be small, and the fried egg should be eaten when quite hot. Boiled eggs should be put first into cold water, and when the water boils the eggs will be cooked enough.

They differ in flavour according to the kind of bird and its food, so that a duck's or goose's egg is stronger than a fowl's egg. The egg of a well-fed barn-door fowl is far sweeter than of one poorly fed, and that of any bird feeding on fish is strong and less agreeable. The egg of the turkey is good and rich, and that of the plover has a very delicate flavour.

Hard-boiled eggs form very good portable food to the traveller, when eaten with bread and butter, and will keep off hunger for a long time. They, however, demand plenty of fluid, and if milk be drunk with them the nourishment will be the greater.

CHAPTER II.

LIQUID FOODS.

MILK.

Milk is the best of all fluid foods, and in nourishment is not unlike meat. It is eaten exclusively by infants, and nothing is more valuable to young children of all ages. As the child grows, bread and other foods are added to the milk, and when he is grown up he eats meat instead of milk.

A young infant needs nothing but the mother's milk, or cow's milk with one-third of warm water and a little sugar. At eight or twelve months old, a little boiled flour may be added to it, and after that time bread, rice, sago, &c., as in making puddings.

Milk is not liked by all persons, but if it be eaten when cooked or hot, and in small quantities, it agrees with almost everybody. Cold milk drank in a large quantity at once often disagrees.

Milk differs very much in flavour and nutriment, according to the food and nature of the cow, so that some specimens have more water, and others more cheese, or butter (Fig. 5). When new it contains water, sugar, cheese, butter, and salts, and has all the kinds of food required by the body. When skimmed it has lost nearly all its butter, but if about half-an-ounce of suet be boiled with a pint of the skimmed milk, or used when making a pudding, it will be nearly equal to new milk. When the cheese as well as the butter have been taken out, the remaining fluid is called whey, and contains water, sugar, acids, and salts, with perhaps a few small lumps of butter, and is therefore valuable, but far less so than either skim-milk or new milk.

When the cream has been churned the butter becomes solid, and is taken out, and only butter-milk is left. This contains some cheese and a little fat or butter, besides sugar, acid, and salts, and is therefore much better than whey, and if not quite equal to skim-milk, is a very good food and should be largely eaten.

In hot weather all these kinds are very agreeable when eaten cold, but in cold weather it is better to warm new and skimmed milk. If milk be boiled, a skin forms upon it, and it is not quite so nourishing. It is sufficient, without boiling it, to make it as warm as it can be drank.

All these are good foods, and none should be thrown away. Some think that skim-milk is worth very little, and butter-milk still less, whilst they give whey (if at all) only to the sick. This is a very great mistake, and the poor should get all the butter-milk and skim-milk they can obtain. If bought they are much cheaper than new milk, and may be purchased when new milk could not be afforded. No doubt new milk is the best of all kinds, and should be obtained for infants and very young children.

Whenever, therefore, a poor man can keep a cow he should do so, both to give milk and butter to his own family and to sell them to others. Many parishes allow cows to feed in the lanes on payment of a small sum weekly, and many landowners and farmers would gladly let cows feed in their fields, on proper payment.

But if a cow cannot be kept, or cow's milk bought, a goat should be obtained, which will give perhaps two quarts of milk a day. The milk is thicker and of stronger flavour than cow's milk, but children will drink it. It should be diluted with one-third or one-half of water.

It is quite certain that the extreme value of milk as a food is not well understood in this country, so that much is given to animals which should be eaten by men, and money is spent upon food of much less value. It is better appreciated in Sweden, Switzerland, and other mountainous countries, for there the men drink several pints daily, and are strong and laborious. Nothing would so much tend to save the life of infants, and to enable children to grow up into healthy men and women, as an abundant use of good milk, and nothing therefore would tend more to lessen disease and mortality.

Its value is, however, the greatest in many states of disease, and particularly in consumption, or the state of weakness which tends to that terrible disease, and the aim should be to take two or three pints daily, either alone or made into puddings.

Every person, whether farmer or consumer, is interested in increasing the supply of milk, and every facility should be offered to the poor to keep cows.

Several remarkable cases of typhoid fever have recently arisen in connection with the use of milk. It is said that even the rinsing of the vessels with foul water has caused it in some, whilst in others the milk has been diluted with such water. Some have affirmed that milk from a house in which there were cases of this fever, has produced it, and that milk allowed to remain in or near a room with them will become poisoned. The influence of foul water in producing the disease is well known, and this may account for the effects of the milk; but whilst care may be taken to avoid milk which comes from a house with typhoid fever, it is impossible for the consumer to know whether the water which is used in the house is perfectly pure or not. The subject deserves the attention of both the producers and the consumers.

WATER.

Water is an indispensable substance for the maintenance of life, and a man entirely without food will live many days longer with, than without, water. It is also found in every kind of food, whether solid or fluid, so that there are about six ounces in every pound of bread, and more than twice that quantity in each pound of fresh meat.

The quantity of water which we eat in our solid foods is not at all generally understood, and therefore the following table will be of interest. In every 100 pounds of foods there is the number of pounds of water to be now stated.

TABLE No. 5.

	lbs.
Sugar	5
Rice	13
Indian Meal	14
Peas, Wheat Flour, Barley Meal, Oatmeal, Rye Meal, Butter and Fats, and Dried Bacon	15
Arrowroot	18
Treacle	23
Green Bacon	24
Cheddar Cheese	36
Bread	37
Fat Pork	39
Skim Milk Cheese	44
Fat Beef	51
Fat Mutton	53
Veal	63
Lean Mutton	72

	lbs.
Egg, Ox Liver	74
Potatoes, Eels	75
Salmon	77
White Fish and White of Egg	78
Parsnips	82
Carrots	83
Turnips	91

In our chief fluid foods there are in a hundred pints the following pints of water:—

	pts.
Cream	66
New Milk	86
Skimmed Milk and Butter Milk	88
Beer and Porter	91

It is of the greatest importance that it be pure, for foul water produces fever and other deadly diseases. If the supply be from water-works, there are people appointed to test its purity. In that case see that the tap and cistern are clean, as also the vessels in which it is kept or carried; but of all these see first to the cistern, and have it covered over and cleaned out three or four times a year.

There are filters which may be placed in the cistern (Fig. 13), and through which all the water may be drawn which is used for drinking or cooking. Filtered water is brighter, clearer, and more agreeable if it be not allowed to remain too long in the filter, and as the cost of filters is now small they should be more generally used. They lose their power after a certain time, but may be readily renovated by the following process:—Take two wine glasses full of Condy's red fluid undiluted, with ten drops of sulphuric acid (oil of vitriol), and a table-spoonful of muriatic acid, and add them to from two to four gallons of water. Then place the whole in the filter for a few hours, after which, pour three gallons of pure soft water through, and it will be ready for use.

If the water is drawn from a well, see that dirty water does not run in at the top, nor any drain, petty, or pigsty be placed so near that filth from it may get into the well. Keep the ground at the top of the well hard and dry, and if possible paved, and keep it lower than the top of the well. Do not let any slops be thrown down near the well. Let the well be covered so that no animal or dirt can fall into it, for a dead cat or rat in the water will do great harm. If possible have a pump instead of a draw-well, and

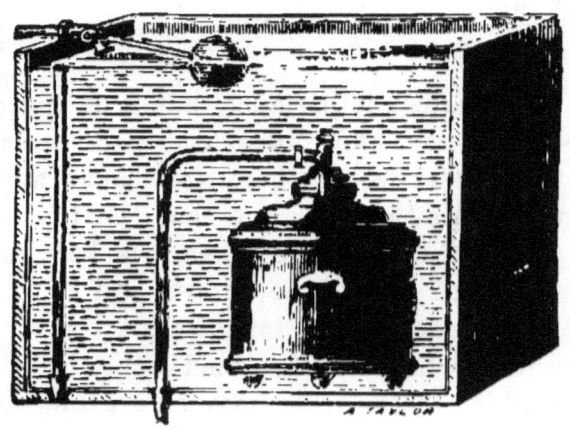

Fig. 13.

FILTER PLACED WITHIN A CISTERN, BY THE LONDON AND GENERAL WATER PURIFYING COMPANY.

if there are any lead pipes, see that the pump is in constant use, or the water may cause lead poisoning. If the water get low in the summer-time, the well should be cleaned out, as the mud at the bottom may do harm.

If water is obtained from a brook see that it is running water, and that there is no filth in it. A filter is easily placed in the brook by making a wooden box, eighteen inches square, and deep enough to be higher than the water. At the bottom, for twelve or eighteen inches in depth, put a quantity of well-burnt bones, crushed or ground very small, and cover them with wood. Bore holes in the side where the burnt bones are for the water from the brook to enter, and also in the cover for the water to go through into the space above, where the filtered water will be stored. The filter should be kept covered.

If the water is not running it is probably not fit for use; but should be boiled and allowed to cool, or be filtered. If any filth goes into it, it should not bo drank.

When water is very hard it wastes a great deal of soap, and it is better to collect rain-water and use it for washing. The cistern should be covered and cleaned out from time to time, for the washings from the roof alone will make it black and leave a deposit. Running water, like brook-water, is the best for making tea, but well-water may be used for cleaning and cooking.

Water should have no smell or taste, and should be perfectly clear and bright. If it have a bad smell or taste it should be examined. If it be not clear, but only muddy from soil washed into it, it will become clear on setting it aside, and may be good water. Such a state of water often occurs in brooks after rains; but when it is clear it should be without taste and smell, like good water, and if otherwise, there is something wrong.

Water should also be cool, as it is then more refreshing in summer; but very cold water sometimes hinders digestion and even causes cramp. When this is so, a little warm water should be added to it to take off the chill.

It is necessary to drink water with solid food, unless some other fluid, as broth, be taken with it, in order that it may be dissolved and distributed, and that other matters which are not needed may be taken out of the system; but it is not well to drink much water at the beginning of the dinner, or to drink at any time more than is needful. There are some people who never drink water alone, because they take enough of other fluids. A man requires two to three pints of some kind of fluid every day, and more in summer than in winter, and with violent exercise than at rest. There are also many substances, as pepper and pickles, taken in food which cause thirst, and induce the eater to drink; and even other fluids, as beer, will add to thirst.

The supply of water to villages is often very deficient both in quantity and quality, and is not only a loss of comfort, but a very frequent cause of disease. Every householder should first see to the water, and wherever a house can be obtained which has a supply from public waterworks, or failing that, from a good deep well, it is worth a higher rental. Diarrhœa or vomiting, especially in hot weather, should lead to an examination of the water, and if there is frequently pain in the bowels, and the water passes through lead pipes, there may be lead poisoning.

TEA AND COFFEE.

If the tea be pure, a cheap kind is as good as an expensive one, for they are all from the same tree, and the only difference is in the flavour. Black and green teas are the same, except that the green is the very young leaf, and contains more of the property of tea. A less quantity of green tea will therefore suffice. The weight of a teaspoonful of different kinds of tea differs very much, and a teaspoonful of green tea is much heavier than one of common black tea. This is of importance in forming a judgment of the qualities and prices of teas, and shows that a small quantity, by measure, of one kind contains really as much as a larger quantity of another kind. This is shown in the following table:—

WEIGHT OF TEAS.

TABLE No. 6.

Black Teas.

	Weight of a Spoonful in Grains.	Number of Spoonfuls in a Pound.
Oolong	39	179
Congou (inferior quality)	52	138
Flowery Pekoe	62	113
Souchong	70	100
Congou (fine)	87	80

Green Teas.

Hyson Skin	58	120
Twankay	70	100
Hyson	66	106
Imperial (fine)	90	77
Caper (scented)	103	68
Gunpowder (fine)	123	57

The quality of tea as it is drank varies not only with the weight of the tea, but with the mode in which it is prepared. When made from hard water, in a cold teapot, with the water not then boiling, and allowed to stand in the cold, good tea cannot be expected. The proper mode of making it is very simple, and yet it is very generally neglected. It is as follows:—

1. Use sufficient tea.
2. Make the pot warm with hot water, or otherwise, before the tea is put into it, or it will cool the hot water.
3. Let the water be boiling at the moment of using it. Water rapidly cools when taken off the fire.
4. Fill up the pot at once.
5. Do not use water which has already been boiled, but boil it fresh for the purpose.
6. Cover the teapot, or place it where it will be kept

nearly as hot as boiling water. Do not place it on iron which is nearly cold—as a cold hob, or fender, or fire-irons—and imagine that it will be kept warm because it is before the fire, for iron draws out the heat very rapidly.

7. Let it stand for ten minutes.

8. Use brook or running water if possible, and it is worth while to take the trouble to obtain a little for that purpose. If well-water be used, or if the water be hard, add a very small pinch of carbonate of soda.

Tea is still very much adulterated, but not so generally as it was some years ago. Other leaves, as those of the sloe-tree, are commonly added; but if you will take a leaf of tea which has been washed and compare it with the others, you will be able to detect the difference. Stalks are often found in the cheaper teas, and if they belong to the leaf they are not without value, but they are not so good as the leaf, and should not be allowed in any considerable quantity. Green teas are sometimes faced with copper so as to make them look bright. Never buy a bright-looking tea. China clay and many other things are added, and even iron filings, to increase the weight, but all these can be ascertained with a little care. Whatever is heavier than leaves will fall to the bottom of the pot.

Some so-called tea does not contain a particle of tea. Thus one quantity is mentioned as consisting wholly of the following substances:—Iron filings, plumbago, chalk, china clay, sand, Prussian blue, turmeric, indigo, starch, gypsum, catechu and gum, and the leaves of the camellia, savanqua, chloranthus, elm, oak, willow, poplar, elder, beech, hawthorn, and sloe.

Tea, even when good, contains very little nutriment—none whatever in proportion to its cost—and therefore there is the more reason for detecting adulterations. It was not known to our forefathers, and they lived well without it, and it is possible that we waste too much money upon it. At the same time we need a warm, agreeable fluid with our meals, and cannot always get milk (which is so much more valuable), or, if we had it, we could not always take the same kind of fluid, and therefore tea has its use. It is, however, a sort of nervous stimulant, for it makes our minds clearer and brighter, and after taking it we are more ready to work.

If, therefore, it is scarcely a food in itself, it helps to quicken the use of good food, and gives us a sense of comfort. It is more fitted for those who eat too much than for the starving, and after a good meal than in place of a meal; and, on the whole, those who have too little food would spend their money much better by buying milk.

Some take tea with meat, and call it a tea dinner, or a meat tea, but tea and meat do not seem to agree well together, and although it may be agreeable as a change, none like it constantly.

When too much tea is taken, and there is not sufficient food with it, or when the stomach is inclined to be irritable, it is very apt to cause indigestion. It is doubtful whether any other thing causes so much indigestion amongst the poor, and when that disorder exists tea must not be taken.

Tea is not fit for the use of infants and young children, for they need stronger food, and that which is not so stimulating. Tea seems to be liked most by those who sit much and take little exercise, particularly if they occupy warm and close rooms or workshops, and it is then the most valuable. At the same time those who take much exercise have less need for it, and desire it less. It is easy, therefore, to see whether too little exercise, and hot and close rooms, with much tea, are likely to be so healthful as much exercise with plenty of real food.

Coffee should, if possible, be fresh and finely ground, but when kept ground it should be in a tightly covered tin. It is better to add about one teaspoonful of chicory to four of coffee. The simplest method of making it is to put it into a warm jug, and pour boiling water upon it; then stir it and cover it, and keep it nearly boiling hot for a few minutes. When pouring it off stop the grounds. The chief use of coffee-pots of every kind is to strain the coffee from the grounds. Much warm milk and some sugar should be drunk with the coffee.

Tea and coffee are both drunk so universally that it might be inferred that they are taken indifferently; but although some persons prefer tea, and others coffee, a selection is usually made, so that coffee is drunk at breakfast (as it should be), and tea at the tea meal. As tea tends to increase, and coffee to decrease perspiration, the former is more fitted for hot and close weather, when we do not perspire enough, and the latter for cold, or any kind of weather when the skin is soft, and we too readily perspire.

Both have a stimulating effect upon the brain, and when taken at night may drive away sleep. They may thus be useful if we wish to remain awake for some special duty, and injurious when we ought to sleep. They differ in this respect in different individuals, and perhaps in the same on various occasions; but, as a rule, they should not be taken late at night in any considerable quantity.

The effect of coffee upon the stomach in producing or continuing indigestion is the same as that of tea, but it is reduced if two-thirds of the quantity be hot milk.

Cocoa and chocolate, when made with milk, are really good foods—far better than tea or coffee, although not so cheering to the spirits—and would be much more useful to the poor.

Cocoa-nibs should be boiled in water for several hours in order to extract all that is valuable as food; but prepared cocoa, being finely ground and mixed with sugar, dissolves very readily in boiling water or milk, and the whole may be eaten. Perhaps few foods are so nutritious, or will satisfy the appetite so well, as cocoa and milk, if plenty of cocoa be used, and it is equally good for all ages, classes, and circumstances.

BEER, WINE, AND SPIRITS.

Nothing can be more certain than that these substances are not necessary to persons in health, and whilst they may be taken in small quantities without injury, they are much more frequently injurious than useful. They contain but little that is truly nutriment, and cannot therefore be properly called foods; yet there is some nutritive material in beer and wine. They are drank chiefly for pleasure or from habit, and therefore might be got rid of without any disadvantage; whilst at the same time they are costly, and cause an enormous waste of money amongst the working classes. The cost of two pints of ale daily, viz., 3s. 6d. a week, would well clothe a whole family, whilst little loss of nutriment would occur by omitting the stimulants.

They do not give strength for work in any proportion to their cost, but on the other hand often make people dull, heavy, stupid, and unfit for work. The most severe and continued work can be performed without them, and there are now some millions of people in this country who never taste them. Happy will be the day when they are not drank by any, but particularly by the working man, who finds it difficult to maintain his family. Then will there be less quarrelling, poverty, and crime, and more food, clothing, and education.

They may be properly used as medicines to give appetite to the sick, or to help digestion, or to stimulate the feeble, and should be ordered by the doctor.

Children who are well should never taste them, and will not want them.

It is said that they increase the heat of the body, and therefore are as useful as some other foods; but in the Arctic regions it was proved that the entire exclusion of spirits was necessary in order to retain heat under those extremely unfavourable conditions. Tea was used by Dr. Kane's sailors; but the question is not whether tea was necessary to maintain heat, but whether alcohols were desirable, and it was clearly proved that they were injurious.

The proper position of these fluids is that of luxuries, or poisons, and not of necessaries. As luxuries they may be tolerated by those who like them and can afford them, but they are intolerable when they brutalize the husband and bring want to the wife and family. Recent experience has shown that the consumption of these articles has doubled, without increasing the respectability and comfort of the working classes. Never was there so little work done, and rarely were rent and shop-bills less regularly paid, or the children less educated.

Every child should resist the temptation to drink them, and be a missionary to endeavour to reclaim others from the practice of this folly.

The basis of all improvement in sanitary arrangements, or in education and morals, must be the diminution, if not the cessation, of the use of these articles by the mass of the people.

If any preference is to be given it should be of ordinary beer over spirits, and the latter should be placed entirely at the disposal of the doctor and for sick people.

BEER, WINE, AND SPIRITS.

About 120 millions of money are spent yearly in these substances, and therefore we may well ask whether so large a sum is wisely spent. If we allow that there are 1,000 millions of people in the whole world, and that a 4 lb. loaf of bread could be purchased everywhere for 6*d*., that sum would feed the whole world with ⅔ lb. of bread daily for one month ; or, if we take the populations of Great Britain and Ireland, Canada, North America, France, Germany, Italy, Spain, Portugal, Greece, Russia, and all the states of Europe together, it would give them the same for about four months. It would supply ⅔ lb. of bread daily to every person in Great Britain, North America, and Canada, all the year round.

Consider then if this were saved how much less starvation there might be, how much fewer women and children need to work merely for a living, and how much better the working man's family might be clad and educated. 120 millions a year means about £4 a year for every man, woman and child in this country, so that a family of six persons would save nearly £25 a year—a sum sufficient to make a little fortune.

If all, or nearly all of it be useless, and much of it far worse than useless, should we not induce those who have not too much money to live without them ?

CHAPTER III.

GENERAL QUESTIONS RELATING TO FOODS.

DIGESTIBILITY OF SOLID FOODS.

THE digestibility of various kinds of foods varies very much, as we all infer from our own experience, and as was proved by the experiments of Dr. Beaumont. This physician had a patient, who by a gun-shot wound had an external opening into the stomach through which substances could be introduced and withdrawn. Small silver balls were prepared so that the juices of the stomach could enter them, and being filled with a food were introduced, and allowed to remain until perfectly digested.

The following table contains the results of these experiments, and is of so much value that it should be committed to memory:—

DIGESTION OF FOODS.

TABLE No. 7.

I.—Animal Food.

Food.	Mode of Cooking.	Time required for Digestion.	
		hrs.	min.
Pork	roasted	5	15
Cartilage	boiled	4	15
Ducks	roasted	4	0
Fowls	do.	4	0
Do.	boiled	4	0

DIGESTIBILITY OF SOLID FOODS.

Food.	Mode of Cooking.	Time required for Digestion.	
		hrs.	min.
Beef	fried	4	0
Eggs	do.	3	30
Do.	hard boiled	3	30
Cheese		3	30
Oysters	stewed	3	30
Mutton	roasted	3	15
Do.	boiled	3	0
Beef	roasted	3	0
Do.	boiled	2	45
Chicken	fricasseed	2	45
Lamb	broiled	2	30
Pig (suckling)	roasted	2	30
Goose	do.	2	30
Gelatin	boiled	2	30
Turkey	do.	2	25
Eggs	roasted	2	15
Cod Fish (cured, dry)	boiled	2	0
Ox Liver	broiled	2	0
Brains	boiled	1	45
Venison Steak	broiled	1	30
Salmon Trout	boiled	1	30
Eggs (whipped)	raw	1	30
Tripe (soused)	boiled	1	0
Pig's feet (soused)	do.	1	0

Many will be surprised to find that vegetable food requires even longer time for digestion than animal food.

II.—*Vegetable Food.*

Food.	Mode of Cooking.	Time required for Digestion.	
		hrs.	min.
Cabbage	boiled	4	0
Beetroot	do.	3	45
Turnips	do.	3	30
Potatoes	do.	3	30
Wheaten bread	baked	3	30
Carrot	boiled	3	15
Indian Corn bread	baked	3	15
Do. cake	do.	3	0
Apple-dumpling	boiled	3	0
Potatoes	baked	2	33
Do.	roasted	2	30
Parsnips	boiled	2	30

Food.	Mode of Cooking.	Time required for Digestion.	
		hrs.	min.
Sponge-cake	baked	2	30
Beans	boiled	2	30
Cabbage (pickled)	raw	2	0
Apples (sour and mellow)	do.	2	0
Barley	boiled	2	0
Tapioca	do.	2	0
Sago	do.	1	45
Apples (sweet and mellow)	raw	1	30
Rice	boiled	1	0

CONDIMENTS.

Certain condiments, as salt, are necessary to health, whilst others as pepper, vinegar, and pickles are agreeable and useful when the appetite fails.

About half an ounce of salt is required daily, but as there is salt in bread and other cooked foods we do not need to eat half that quantity by itself. There are some who do not eat salt separately, and who therefore say that they do not eat it at all, but although the quantity required may vary, it is absolutely essential that some should be taken and particularly with vegetables.

Pepper and mustard are useful to give flavour to tasteless foods, and to stimulate the sense of taste and the flow of saliva and gastric juice. They should, however, be taken in moderation, for they may excite indigestion, and after much use simple foods are not enjoyed. So long as ordinary food is eaten and the appetite is good, the use of these things is unnecessary and becomes simply a matter of habit.

Vinegar is often useful as a food, and particularly in hot weather, when we crave for acids, whether in fruits or otherwise, and as meat is less relished in hot than in cold weather, and does not contain acids, we find vinegar and pickles very agreeable and even useful additions to it.

Too much vinegar is, however, very injurious, and by causing indigestion and loss of appetite, makes people thin. Neither pickles nor vinegar are really necessary to those who are well and can obtain various foods according to the season, but on ship-board they are often of the greatest use.

Pickles made very strong with pepper are also much more used in India and other hot countries where the appetite fails than in England.

POISONOUS SUBSTANCES SOMETIMES EATEN.

Many deaths have been caused by eating poisonous mushrooms and puff-balls. It is now said that there are many kinds of mushrooms which may be eaten without danger, but it will be better to eat only the one kind which is known to be not poisonous. They have an agreeable smell and pinkish gills; and those should be preferred which grow in the open field, and not under trees or in a wood. Moreover, the large are not so good as the small. Be sure to smell them, and take care that the gills are not white; and if you have any doubt do not eat them. Many of the very gaily coloured mushrooms are very poisonous. Puff-balls should not be eaten.

Horse chestnuts are not so agreeable in flavour as the Spanish; and they are also acrid and cause pain in the stomach and bowels, like a poison.

The bulbs or roots of the arum, or as they are called "bulls and cows," should not be eaten.

The berries of the mountain-ash are said to be poisonous.

The wild lettuce is poisonous.

The berry of the potato is poisonous.

The black berries of the deadly nightshade in gardens, and of the dulcamara in the hedges, are poisonous.

The root of the aconite or monkshood, which is poisonous, is sometimes mistaken for horse-radish, and is scraped and eaten. The form of the root is not the same in both cases, and the smell and taste are very different. Before eating scraped horse-radish always smell it, and taste a very little.

Two plants, which grow with water-cress in ditches and ponds, are sometimes gathered with it and eaten for it; viz., the veronica and water-parsley, and although not very poisonous are not fit for food. They are distinguished without much difficulty by a slight examination, but when the water-cress has grown to a large size it is less unlike the water-parsley.

Tobacco is sometimes ranked with foods, but can it be beneficial under any circumstances? Many say it can, but we deny it as far as regards people in health. It frequently lessens the appetite, makes the head ache, and weakens the body, which food does not. It contains no nourishment, but, on the contrary, is a powerful poison when the smoke is retained in the body, so powerful that doctors dare not use it. There is much more harm received from smoking than people imagine, and every one in health would be better without it.

It is also a very expensive habit which causes great waste of money and leads to poverty, whilst at the same time it is disagreeable to many and makes clothing and furniture smell very offensively.

It is quite true that many people smoke throughout life and seem none the worse for it, but it is equally true that many others are seriously injured, and unable by reason of it to perform some of the duties of life. No greater foe to the throat and the digestion exists, and many persons by the constant use of it fall into both mental and bodily disease. This is dependent, no doubt, upon the degree in which it is consumed, the quality of the tobacco, the mode of smoking, and the peculiarities of the system, so that in the one it is simply an amusement which leaves little evil behind, whilst in another it is almost the occupation of life, and emasculates both mind and body. Bad tobacco, a foul pipe, and constant smoking, produce disease of the throat.

It may be true that tobacco is smoked with impunity, but it is equally true that the whole tendency of its action is towards disease, and it is impossible to say how much of good it has prevented. When to this is added the nuisance which it creates to many, the waste of money which might have been profitably employed, and which was perhaps needed for education or other modes of advancement in life, or for the help of those nearly related, it can be regarded as little less than a sin, and we might regret that the habit was ever acquired. But it is "never too late to mend." Those who have been inveterate smokers have under a sense of responsibility broken off the habit. We would earnestly counsel those who do not smoke tobacco never to acquire the habit, and those who do smoke to make better use of their money, time, and nervous power.

It is, doubtless, a delusion to believe that the mind is more fitted for work when soothed by tobacco. Without referring to states of disease which are exceptional, we are of opinion that it is more fitted to discharge the duties of life when not under the influence of this or any other narcotic.

Tobacco is made from a handsome-looking plant which grows to the height of six feet. The leaves are large, soft, and of a dark green colour, whilst the flower is red, and when seen in great masses is a very pretty object. The plant is not cultivated in this country for the manufacture of tobacco on account of the great tax which is levied upon tobacco by the government, but is grown as an ornament in our flower gardens, and the leaves are sometimes dried to be used by gardeners in killing insects by smoke.

The cultivation and preparation of this substance occupies great numbers of persons in America and the Spanish colonies, and the capital and enterprise involved may bear some relation to the production of wine. Even the selection of the leaves for the kinds of tobacco demands great skill and knowledge of the market; and delicacy of taste in the selection of tobaccos grown in different soils and in various climates is as essential as it is to a tea-taster or a wine merchant. The great variety which the tobacconist offers to his customer depends upon, firstly, soil and climate; secondly, selection and preparation; and thirdly, admixture of the leaves of other plants, and the addition of substances to give strength and flavour.

It seems simple to say that tobacco is the dried leaf of the tobacco-plant, and should have one quality, but few preparations are more complicated by questions of selection, flavour, and names. It must be ranked with luxuries, and not with necessaries, whether food or medicine.

HINTS ABOUT COOKING.

We have already referred to cooking under three of the heads of foods, but it is desirable to consider the subject in a somewhat more general manner, for on the right mode will depend the healthfulness and the economy of the food to be eaten.

The object of cooking should be well understood, and then the methods employed will be better appreciated. It is not to change the food, for a potato is almost precisely the same after as before boiling, but to make it more tender, so that it may be easily broken up by the teeth, to improve its flavour, and to supply warmth to the body.

The first requirement is perfect cleanliness, so that no foreign substance may be added to the food, and that the eater may not be disgusted. This implies clean saucepans, basins, knives, forks, and spoons, and all other utensils—clean hands, clean clothes, and good habits in handling and tasting food. This is not found in England as it should be, or even as it exists in France. In the latter country nearly all their saucepans and other metal utensils are made of copper, which are kept bright on the outside, and in the inside are tinned and retinned from time to time. Ours are generally of iron, which are very greasy on the outside, and dark and discoloured on the inside; and though the inside may be as clean as hot water can make it, it does not look so. One might eat food in a French saucepan, but not in an English one. This is partly due to the different kind of fuel which is used, for in France it is charcoal, which gives very little smoke, and in England it is coal, which deposits soot on everything it touches.

Scrape the outside of the saucepan and frying-pan, and scour the inside as well as wash it well in boiling water, and do not leave the handle so greasy that it should digust you to use it. Make all those utensils which are liable to be dirty really clean, and look clean.

A newly-tinned saucepan is not very healthful, for some of the solder acts upon the water and food, and may give colic. It is better to boil some bran and water, or potato-peelings and water in it, and to throw them away before using it for cooking, or to place it in hot water for a day. If the vessel be of copper, the tinning should be renewed as it is wanted, or the copper will injure the food; but with iron vessels it is of less importance. Never boil anything, and particularly acid foods like fruits, in an untinned copper vessel.

As certain foods, as milk, are apt to burn when placed upon the fire, and to adhere to the sides of the saucepan, care should be taken to clean the vessel before it is again used for cooking.

If cooking-forks be dirty between the prongs and left so after use, they will injure the flavour of the food. Keep knives, forks, and spoons which are used in cooking as clean and bright as those used in eating.

Crockery and glass, whether good or common, are often very imperfectly washed in greasy water, which is not thoroughly wiped off. Teacups show marks of food outside, and neither the inside nor outside is bright and shining. They should always be well washed and rinsed in clean hot water, and after being drained, should be well dried and polished with a dry towel.

Dirty and greasy hands are an abomination in a cook, for she must handle some foods as they are moved about, and people must eat the dirt. It is no doubt difficult to keep the hands clean, but it is much less so to one who is careful to use forks and spoons, and who appreciates the fact that some one must eat what she has handled. Many handle bread, meat, butter, cheese, and nearly every kind of food needlessly, and should be taught to use clean forks and spoons. Matters which are not only offensive and disgusting, but really prejudicial to health, may be conveyed by dirty hands. When her hands are dirty, she may wash them with a loss of two minutes only.

It is necessary in making soups and other dishes to taste the food from time to time in order to judge as to the flavour, and not unfrequently the same spoon which conveyed the food to the mouth, is put back into the dish or saucepan, and used again and again. This is a dirty habit, and it is better to take out a small quantity of the soup with one spoon, and taste of it with another.

Dirty aprons and dirty handles will certainly make dirty hands, and dirty, greasy dish-cloths and towels will not make clean dishes and clean food.

When food is to be boiled, the vessel should be placed upon a bright fire, and not thrust into the smoke as though it were intended to foul both the food and the vessel. Smoked milk, broth, or tea, is very disagreeable, and smoked vessels require to be cleaned. A small red fire will cook better than a large, black, smoky one, and a furnace which can be closed so that the saucepan may be placed on the hot plate, will be far more cleanly and less troublesome.

The oven should not be too hot. No food should be placed in one which is red hot on one side, for it will be burnt on that side before it is warmed through on the other. Let the temperature be nearly the same on all sides, and take care to regulate the heat by the right use of the dampers. It is also desirable to see that there is an opening through which the steam may escape, or the food may be sodden, but in even the best range it is desirable to open the door occasionally to examine and turn the food, and to allow the steam to escape.

Cooking-ranges vary much in fitness and economy, but many may now be obtained which burn little fuel in proportion to the heat produced, and which allow the heat to be well regulated.

Gas-stoves also claim attention, for they distribute the heat more uniformly and cleanly, and may be more economical than coal-grates if properly regulated. **They are** lighted and extinguished instantly, and therefore need be used only when required, and are employed in nearly all large establishments in towns. Objection was formerly taken to the flavour of the meat thus roasted, but now that the stoves are lined with clay or terra-cotta, they are unobjectionable.

There are but few foods which require to be cooked in boiling water, for they will be better cooked in water below that heat, say at 180° F. This is the case with meat, milk, eggs, and soup, and the reason is that the albumen (like the white of egg) becomes solid at 180°, and hard and less digestible at the boiling point. Therefore meat kept at 180° will be tender and digestible, whilst, boiled at 212°, it will be hard and almost indigestible. It may be that the cook has no thermometer, but she knows when fluid is kept under the boiling point, and therefore below 212°, and may readily guess that it is sufficiently near that heat.

The use of the Norwegian-stove is in this respect as well as for economy very good. It is simply a box lined with felt four to six inches in thickness, and when a vessel containing boiling water is placed in it and closed up, it will keep it hot enough during the whole time required for cooking food. Thus if a leg of mutton be placed in a vessel with boiling water and just boiled on the fire, it may be enclosed in the box whilst the housewife attends to other duties; and without further expense for fuel or further attention will be found cooked at the proper time. This arrangement is very simple, cleanly, and economical, and any one may make such a box for a few shillings. Let some child explain this to her mother and induce her to try it, and particularly in those parts of the country where fuel is very dear.

Milk, soup, tea and coffee should not be boiled, but tea

and coffee should be made with boiling water poured into a pot which has already been made quite hot, and then kept quite warm.

Fresh vegetables require more heat than the substances already named, but when once boiled they may be allowed to simmer. Care should be taken to cook them well, but they should not be boiled down lest the flavour should be lessened and waste caused.

Much attention is required to roast meat, whether before the fire or in a stove, so that it shall be done throughout, and yet the juices be retained within it. Not unfrequently it is underdone or overdone, and few can eat the former, whilst the latter causes waste of food. It should be dried on the outside quickly, and then exposed to a lower heat. Veal and pork require more cooking than beef or mutton, for they are less agreeable and digestible when underdone, and therefore there is often much waste.

Bread does not require this management, but should be baked at an even temperature throughout; but pies containing meat will often be cooked on the outside before the inside is ready for the table, unless the meat be previously in part cooked; and if the inside consist of several substances, as meat and potato, the difficulty becomes greater. A good cook will take care that all are equally cooked when eaten.

The flavour of nearly every food is changed and improved when cooked, but persons differ as to the degree in which they would have food cooked. Thus some prefer a piece of beef which is red and full of juice, and others the outside which is dried and has the flavour of burnt flesh. Hence, there is no universal rule, but each household must have its own law. At the same time a perfectly roasted joint will supply both kinds, at least to a limited extent, for the outer part will be more cooked than the inner. A joint which is undercooked and remains raw and sodden is rarely liked, and the less so if it be served in a half-cold state.

The digestibility of foods varies with the mode and degree of cooking, as has been already proved by Dr. Beaumont's experiments, but it also varies with the temperature at which it is eaten. Cold foods rarely digest so well as when hot, particularly in old persons; whilst a half-cooked joint served up lukewarm is still less digestible. Hence it is desirable that food should be properly cooked and then served when as warm as it can be conveniently eaten.

The warming-up of food also demands a passing remark, for it may over-cook the food by excessive heat, and make that hard and tough which at the first cooking was tender. If it be undesirable to boil meat at first it is equally so in warming it up in stews.

The subject of waste is intimately connected with cooking.

Loss of weight of meat is not necessarily waste, for nearly all except water may be retained, and the quantity which remains will afford as much nutriment as the larger quantity before cooking. If, however, the lean or the fat be burnt or too much cooked there will be a real loss. Boiled meat should lose about one-fourth of its weight, and that which is removed should be found in the broth, whilst roasted meat will lose about one-third besides the weight of the dripping. Many cooks, however, throw away the broth, or dirty or sell the dripping, all of which is improper.

Bones should not be roasted, if they can be removed from the meat, but boiled. If broken or sawn into small pieces, and then placed with water in a digester with a lid which is fastened down, and stewed for twelve to twenty-four hours, they will afford very valuable material with which to help to make soup. Every thrifty housewife should not only save the bones but buy others for this purpose. This is a part of cookery and feeding with which we are not sufficiently familiar in this country, but the high price of meat should teach us to be more economical.

Cooked food of every kind should be placed where there is fresh, pure, and cool air, and where insects cannot deposit their eggs upon it. The power of absorption of gases and liquids, which is possessed by both cooked and uncooked food is insufficiently appreciated, or better larders would be provided in good houses. Under present arrangements there is no part of a house for any class in towns which is so defective, but in the country nearly all the better class of houses have cellars which are cool. The air should, moreover, be dry and in motion. Moist and stagnant air is most conducive to putrefaction and particularly in hot and close weather, whilst air which is in motion is generally cool and comparatively dry. Take care, therefore, that there is a good pantry or cellar, that it is well drained, and has a strong current of air passing through it. Do not place the food near any drain, water-closet, or any other source of offensive smells, nor in a close cupboard containing a variety of things and near a fire. Cover it in warm weather in such a manner that flies may be excluded whilst air is admitted, and watch it from time to time.

CHAPTER IV.

CLOTHING.

The requisite clothing depends upon the coldness of the weather, and as we live in a very variable climate the necessary amount varies more than daily.

1. As to the underclothing. Linen next the skin very readily gives a sensation of cold after the body has been heated and has perspired, so that it rather tends to give than to prevent colds. Calico absorbs a larger quantity of moisture and is much warmer under the same circumstances, but woollen whilst it absorbs less is the warmest of all. As the skin perspires in hot weather it is not desirable to wear linen next it, and calico or woollen should be substituted according to the heat of the weather. In cold or cool weather there can be no doubt that woollen is preferable, but in the heat of summer calico may be substituted. In our climate we are, however, liable to chilly evenings with warm days, and a thin woollen vest is safer than an extra calico shirt.

Woollen vests for cold weather may be either thick woven Scotch shirts, or made of fine Welsh flannel. Fitting the body is, however, quite as important as closeness of texture, for if they do not fit well the cold air will find access underneath it. Hence the woven shirt is often a better protector than flannel, but the texture should be close. This is also the case when in any weather much exertion is followed by rest, in which latter state cold may be readily taken. In warm weather a thinner wool, as that of merino, may be substituted, and unless the weather be very hot it is generally the proper clothing.

In this respect, however, persons differ, as they do or do not perspire readily, and as their skins are sensitive; for he who perspires readily requires woollen to prevent cold, whilst a dry and hot skin may be sufficiently protected by calico clothing.

It is much to be regretted that women do not always wear woollen next the skin, whether in summer or winter; and still more so, that there are men who are much exposed to cold, and do not wear it. All persons should wear it from their infancy.

2. As to outer clothing. It is necessary that there should be an outer garment which may be worn or thrown off according to the weather and the sensation of heat. This may be a cloak, coat, or shawl; and provided the trunk be covered, the arms and legs may be covered or uncovered. This should be of woollen, even for women, and even in warm weather.

3. The intermediate clothing. This must depend upon the means of the wearer, mode of life, and season. In cold weather it should no doubt be of wool, whether for women or men; but at other seasons calico and silk may be substituted for women, and perhaps linen for men. The very proper tendency of our day is, however, in favour of wearing woollen fabrics for outdoor wear by both sexes, and at almost all seasons; but in the hot season they are exceedingly light, and of open texture. They are also the most economical, and, as now manufactured, look extremely well. How much better does a good woollen dress look than a dirty and crushed calico, and in the end how much cheaper!

Hence, at all seasons, and for every kind of clothing for outdoor wear, woollen is to be preferred.

When silk or very light fabrics are worn by women there should be sufficient underclothing, besides the woollen vest.

Clothing in the house must necessarily differ from that for outdoor at the same season, but the difference should be chiefly in the outer garment.

There are few if any subjects so important in the management of children as clothing, to protect them from changes of temperature; and both for them and for the old it is desirable that it should be such as shall not oppress by heat or starve with cold. Too much clothing, by causing the skin to perspire freely, makes them more liable to take colds, whilst undue cold lessens vitality. Persons in middle life are more able to resist these as all other influences.

Clothing at night is also worthy of attention. A thick and heavy cotton counterpane weighs down the body without giving much warmth, so that the body is working during sleep, and is less refreshed in the morning. Except the sheets, all coverings of the bed should be of wool, which gives the greatest warmth in proportion to its weight, and the counterpane should be either equal to a blanket, or a blanket should be substituted for it, and a thin light covering like a sheet thrown over it. If there be too much warmth the body is relaxed, the skin made sensitive, and health is impaired. If too little warmth, the body is unnecessarily wasted by loss of heat. The old rule is, however, a good one—viz., to keep the feet warm and the head cool.

Hence, the number of blankets to be used must vary with the weather and season.

Young children and old people need more clothing at night than those of middle age, and in winter the most is required, for all ages, at about four to six o'clock in the morning, when the cold is the greatest. The sick demand great consideration in this matter, and usually need more clothing than those who are well.

What kind of night-dress should be worn? Some say a calico covered by a woollen dress, and others calico only. The very young and aged should have the former, and those of middle age the latter; but if there be rheumatism about the shoulders, it is better to wear the former, and to cover the arms. With such a woollen dress fewer blankets will be required.

In travelling, and when making very varying degrees of exertion, it is desirable to carry a Scotch plaid shawl of fine wool, which is both light and warm, and may be used by night or day, and over any part of the body.

Woollen stockings are desirable for persons with cold feet, and are perhaps better than cotton for everybody; and shoes or boots, strong and thick, according to the season and work, should be worn.

Especial care should be taken as to the clothing of infants and very old people in cold weather, for the absence of a sufficient degree of heat often causes death. It need not entirely cover the face of infants, as we sometimes see, for then they could scarcely breathe, and are liable to suffocation; but it is desirable that such young creatures should not breathe extremely cold air. In reference to the aged, great attention should be paid to the warmth of their extremities, for the circulation being feeble and the production of heat small, the hands and feet may become cold, and exhaustion, leading to death, may result.

Nothing but flannel or some other woollen clothing can be sufficient protection to either of these classes, and much injury results from the absence of it.

CHAPTER V.

MOVEMENTS OF THE BODY.

EXERTION.

EXERTION, whether called labour, recreation, or amusement, is essential to health, and as the body was made for labour, work is its natural and honourable duty.

An idle man or woman is a discredit to the race, and unusually liable to fall into disease, whilst an industrious person adds to the wealth of the country, and is more likely to be healthy and happy.

Exertion is useful, inasmuch as it quickens the circulation, deepens and quickens the breathing, promotes perspiration, and stimulates digestion, and thus helps the body to take food, and to get rid of that which is not required. This is so marked, that the breathing is seven times more with fast running than when lying down at rest. The pulse is quicker when sitting than lying, when standing than sitting, when walking than standing, and when running in proportion to the speed. Even moving the hand affects these actions.

This subject is so interesting that I will introduce the results of a very large series of experiments which I made as to the influence of nearly all kinds of exertion:—

Table No. 8.

Effect of Exertion.

The lying posture . . . . being	1
The sitting posture . . . . is	1·18
Reading aloud or singing . . . . . . ,,	1·26
The standing posture . . . . . . ,,	1·33
Railway travelling in the 1st class . . . . ,,	1·40
,, ,, ,, 2nd class . . . . ,,	1·5
,, ,, upon the engine, at 20 to 30 miles per hour ,,	1·52
,, ,, ,, 50 to 60 ,, ,, ,,	1·55
,, ,, in the 3rd class . . . . . ,,	1·58
,, ,, upon the engine, average of all speeds . ,,	1·58
,, ,, ,, at 40 to 50 miles per hour ,,	1·61
,, ,, ,, 30 to 40 ,, ,, ,,	1·64
Walking in the sea . . . . ,,	1·65
,, on land at 1 mile per hour . . . . . ,,	1·9
Riding on horseback at the walking pace . . . . ,,	2·2
Walking at 2 miles per hour . . . . . . ,,	2·76
Riding on horseback at the cantering pace . . . ,,	3·16
Walking at 3 miles per hour . . . . . . ,,	3·22
Riding moderately . . . . ,,	3·33
Descending steps at 640 yards perpendicular per hour . ,,	3·43
Walking at 3 miles per hour and carrying 34 lbs. . ,,	3·5
,, ,, ,, ,, ,, 62 ,, . ,,	3·84
Riding on horseback at the trotting pace . . . ,,	4·05
Swimming at good speed . . . . . . ,,	4·33
Ascending steps at 640 yards perpendicular per hour . ,,	4·4
Walking at 3 miles per hour and carrying 118 lbs. . ,,	4·75
,, 4 miles per hour . . . . . ,,	5·0
The tread-wheel, ascending 45 steps per minute . . ,,	5·5
Running at 6 miles per hour . . . . . ,,	7·0

The reason why exertion is beneficial by increasing the vital actions is, that the greater the action within the body, the more food is consumed, and the higher the health, (if it be natural and there be sufficient food,) whilst with sloth there is less vital action, and less health.

There is a restriction, however, as to exertion, for the breathing and pulsation are limited in frequency to a point beyond which life cannot be maintained. This limit varies in different persons, and according to practice and habit, so that one man can do that which is impossible to another. But the greater the exertion, the stronger and larger are the muscles which make it, so that the blacksmith's arm is much larger than that of an idle man. Thus, the more you do, the more you will be able to do.

The best time to make great exertion is about two hours after a meal. It is not a good time before breakfast, although moderate work may be then performed; and those who go to work before breakfast should first take a cup of hot milk, tea, or coffee, or other simple food. The body is weakest before breakfast.

After a full meal it is not good to take any violent exercise, but ordinary work may then be properly performed. After the labour of the day, the body becomes tired, and therefore the evening is not the best time for work.

Some persons work all night, but it is not so healthful as working by day. It is easier to work in cool weather than in hot, but in excessively cold weather the limbs are benumbed, and cannot move so readily. In hot weather the most laborious work should be done in the morning and evening, and light work in the middle of the day.

Increase of food is required with much work. If the appetite fail, the body becomes weak; but if it remain good, the body is strengthened. Therefore, in the healthy state, the appetite indicates the quantity of food which is required.

Women are not able to do heavy work like men, because their bones and muscles are not so large, but they do light and delicate work better. Children should not be required to make great exertion, as their bones are not solid at the ends. Old men cannot make so much exertion as the young or the middle-aged, and their bones are more brittle and liable to be broken. An old woman of eighty years of age falling down, is very liable to break her thigh at the hip joint.

Violent or rapid exertion made by children, and also by stout or aged people, often injures, and sometimes causes disease of the heart, when the same taken in the ordinary way would do no harm. Rapidly running up-stairs, or to meet a train, sometimes causes death. Hence, whilst exercise is of the utmost importance to health, it should be taken in a regulated and rational manner, and particularly by those who have passed the period of youth. But disease of the heart even in youth may often be traced to indiscretion in this particular, whether in rowing, running, or jumping.

The kinds of exercise will be further referred to under the heads of "Occupation," "Recreation," and "Gymnastics."

OCCUPATION.

There are perhaps more occupations that are unfavourable than favourable to health, and all need to be watched lest they should lessen health.

Persons who sit at desks or work in close rooms, as clerks, teachers, printers, tailors, and shoemakers, are liable to diseases from want of bodily exercise, and from foul air. Those who bend the body forward, have the chest flattened or contracted. Plumbers are liable to colic from the lead which they use. Match-makers are injured by the phosphorus; chimney-sweeps by the soot; millers, grinders, and those who work in dust, breathe it, and get disease of the chest. Colliers are liable to explosions in the coal-pits, and miners generally, often breathe very foul air. Farm labourers, who so often wear wet clothes, are liable to rheumatism; and all persons are liable to accidents in pursuing their occupations.

It is desirable that each person should know his own

danger and try to prevent it, or to remedy any injuries caused by it.

Thus those who sit much should walk about when they can do so, and after working hours take plenty of exercise in the open air.

Those who stand much should sit when possible.

Those who bend forward should try to sit or stand more upright, and when their work is over they should throw their arms back, stand upright, open the chest, and breathe deeply, and thus try to expand the chest. When they walk they should be upright and keep their shoulders back, and the deeper they breathe, as in running, the more they will expand and open the chest. It is quite possible to prevent any injury from such work by proper care when work is over. The two evils now mentioned apply to women and children, and to a greater number of young men than any other, and hence, wherever there is a gymnasium, or any place where gymnastics can be performed, they should attend. In both these cases there is also a tendency to want of appetite, insufficient food, and indigestion, and the health fails because there is not much exertion made, and the air which they breathe is usually warm and foul. Proper exercise will remedy these evils, at least to a great extent, if the person appreciates the danger to which he is exposed and will diligently try the remedy.

Other trades, as those of plumbers and chimney-sweeps, require that the skin shall not be needlessly covered with paint or soot, and that the hands and face shall be well washed several times a day.

Those who breathe dust should wear a piece of fine gauze, with or without cotton wool, over the mouth and nose, by which some of it will be kept out of the lungs, and every means should be taken to prevent it, and to remove it from the room by good ventilation. The two latter are the most important, since they may be the most effectual; but those who are obliged to be very near the place where dust is made—as steel grinders—should wear the gauze and cotton wool, even when there is good ventilation and a fan is used in the workshop.

There would be fewer explosions in coal and other mines, and fewer deaths from foul air, if the miners would use proper precautions. All should take care that the laws are obeyed, and report any one who, by breaking them, may cause the death of others. The miners themselves must be their own protectors.

There would be much less rheumatism if people were more careful to avoid the rain and to change their wet clothes for dry ones. This is no doubt difficult or even impossible with some, but it is possible with many; and thousands of poor labourers, who can no longer work because of rheumatism, might now maintain their families, if they had contrived to keep old dry clothes to wear when the others were wet. So also the bed and bedclothes should be dry, and no person should knowingly sleep in a damp bed or sit in damp clothes.

Let each person ascertain the particular danger to which he is exposed, and use common sense when trying to prevent it, and he will very generally succeed.

The ventilation of workshops is of the utmost moment, and yet it is very little attended to. The rooms are generally overcrowded, whilst there are noxious fumes from gas burners or charcoal stoves, which are very likely to bring on, or increase, diseases of the throat and chest. They are also almost always too hot, and thereby make the workmen and workwomen more likely to take colds, become feeble, and fall into consumption.

Many good laws have been passed to regulate these questions in factories, workshops, brickyards, furnaces, and other places, and the workmen should see that they are properly carried out. Tailors' shops, printing offices, and milliners' rooms in towns, are very unhealthy, whilst cotton mills are generally too warm. Such workpeople should carry over-clothing to be put on when they leave the mill or workshop, to prevent colds.

Children are now very properly forbidden to work in such unhealthy places, and thereby an opportunity is given them to grow up healthy and strong before they enter on the duties of life; and the hours of labour for all classes have been restricted of late years, so that less injury may be inflicted. All these laws are intended for the protection of the working people, to improve their health, and to prevent fevers, consumption, and other diseases. Special inspectors are appointed by the Government to watch their operation, and the workmen should call their attention to any infringement of them.

RECREATION.

Recreation is necessary in order to maintain health of body. This differs with the circumstances of each person and the period of life, but in some degree and of some kind it is desirable for all.

It may be said that bodily recreation is not needful for a working man who makes enough exertion without it, but that is not correct. Different kinds of work cause certain classes of muscles to act, but not all of them, and recreation, by giving more variety of action, calls the latter into play. A hard-working man even may find recreation and health in a bodily sense, in a game of cricket. But work is not always hard, and a very large proportion of working men and women sit or stand during their labour, and do not make great exertion. They, therefore, above all others, need to engage in exercise or recreation to bring all their muscles into play. So also richer people who are not required to do much bodily work need recreation. There is also a larger class of people who work with their brains, and not with their bodies, and who become very tired and exhausted at the end of the day. They are usually the least inclined to take recreation, and yet they greatly need it daily.

Hence there is no man, woman, or child, whether rich or poor, idle or industrious, who would not be the better for recreation. But even so good a thing should be used with reasonable caution; for as it is clear that work is our first duty, and that no one could be justified in neglecting it, recreation should, therefore, be limited to suitable times and places. It should not be taken with a view to evade work, but to lessen the evil effects of it, and to keep the body well fitted for duty. Recreation which leads to idleness will tend to vice, poverty, and disease, and not to health, and is not that which we recommend. So, also, it should be enjoyed under proper conditions of weather, so that colds may not be taken, or clothing unduly injured; and without evil influences, undesirable associates, foul language, and intoxicating drinks. If it lead to waste and drunkenness it is an evil, and not a good.

Therefore each person should select the kind of recreation, and the time and circumstances, which best suit his requirements and convenience, and always remember that more harm may be obtained from evil associates and habits, at play than at work.

The recreation to which we refer is, however, chiefly of

the out-door kind, such as walking, running, jumping, batting and foot-ball, and the many kinds known to both boys and men in this country. Girls cannot engage in many of these, but they may select such as require running and walking, and will be the more healthy for such kinds of exertion.

Even such well-known kinds of recreation require regulation, so that we may learn to stand, walk, run, skip, and jump in the best way, with a view to perfectly develope the powers of the body, and this is the object of the science of Gymnastics.

GYMNASTICS.

Some kinds of gymnastic exercises are performed in nearly every school of this country, and it is desirable that the practice should be extended and become universal. There is, however, a general approval of them, without sufficiently recognising their importance or appreciating the precise object which should be had in view.

In their utilitarian aspect the object is to develope every class of muscles, to make the body more agile, and to teach certain movements which, under special circumstances, may be most useful, and as a necessary consequence to get rid of superfluous water and fat from the body by exciting all vital actions, particularly those of the skin and lungs.

Regarded as an amusement, they have the advantages just indicated, besides those of spending an hour agreeably and of withdrawing the attention from other amusements of a less desirable nature.

But, however useful and entertaining, they require to be practised with judgment and moderation, for it is as possible to over-excite the functions and organs of the body as those of the heart and skin, and by excess to induce exhaustion and disease rather than health.

The scheme as carried out in our best gymnasiums, for example, that at Oxford, under the able guidance of Mr. MacLaren, is very extensive, and by graduation according to practice and ability is very complete, and is based upon the model of the French, which has been long in operation as a system of training for the army. It includes the following: Walking, running, leaping, climbing, and the use of the leaping-rope, leaping-pole, horizontal beam, vaulting bar, vaulting horse, fixed parallel bars, movable parallel bars, trapezium, pair of rings, row of rings, elastic ladder, horizontal bar, bridge ladder, plank, ladder plank, inclined ladder, prepared wall, vertical pole, fixed vertical pole, slanting pole, turning pole, pair of vertical poles, pair of slanting poles, vertical rope, rotary and mast.

This is a very long array of means for the development of the muscles, and to attain perfect agility. The whole scheme is doubtless desirable for those who would perfect themselves, but it cannot be said to be necessary for the attainment of health and strength, or for the masses of the people. Whilst, therefore, we would advise the use of as many as may be within reach (in due subjection to strength and leisure), it will suffice for our purpose if we indicate the simpler ones, which are now or may soon be found in our ordinary schools. We will, however, further premise that the whole scheme is divided into several classes, according to practice, so that the simpler occupy the first course, and the more difficult the second, third, and fourth courses.

Those of the first course, under Mr. MacLaren's instructions, are as follows:—

1. To walk, at slow time, a short distance.
2. To run, at slow time, a short distance.

3. To leap height, in one or two movements, when standing;—

To leap width.

4. The same, when running.
5. To leap height and width with the rope.
6. To leap width standing with the pole.
7. The front, rear, and side march, when sitting, with the horizontal beam.
8. The same, when upright.
9. To vault over the bar in three movements.
10. To vault over the horse, in one or two movements, when standing;—

To vault over the horse.

11. The same, when running.
12. The single and double march backwards and forwards, on the fixed parallel bars, when travelling.
13. To clear the bar by the front when oscillating.

To rest on the left bar and clear the right by the front.

14. To clear the movable bars, resting on the first or second, over the bars.

To pass from the first to the second bar, with either hand leading, under the bars.

To rest on the single and double bars between the bars.

15. To rise by the single rope, or both ropes, or the back-lift of the trapezium.
16. To make the single and double circle with a pair of rings, and to turn with the feet in the rings.
17. The swing.
18. Travelling on the horizontal bar, with either hand leading, sideways, and with the legs bent or pending.

Rising to the bar three times with the hands direct or reversed.

GYMNASTICS. 85

19. The bridge ladder, by the sides, with either hand leading backwards or forwards.
20. The plank, with hands and feet, and either hand, side, or foot leading.
21. The same, with the ladder plank, backwards or forwards.
22. The same, with the inclined ladder, and above the ladder.
23. The same, with the prepared wall.
24. The vertical pole with hands and feet, either hand leading, or hand over hand.
25. The same, with the slanting pole, both above and under the pole.
26. The turning pole, with either hand leading.
27. The same, with a pair of slanting poles.
28. The vertical rope, with hands and feet, either hand leading, and with the foot in the half turn, full turn, or in the stirrup loop.
29. The simple climb.

We will now very shortly describe those which are in general use, and may be taught in all schools.

THE SINGLE HORIZONTAL POLE.

This may be supported at one or both ends, and should be a few inches above the reach of a person standing on tiptoe. It may be either fixed, or suspended and movable.

1. Jump up and seize the pole with the thumb and fingers on the upper side, and hang by the fingers. (Fig. 14.)
2. Move along the pole backwards and forwards by moving the hands. (Fig. 14.)
3. Draw yourself up slowly until your chest is on a level with the pole, and then suddenly rise to the full height of

the straightened arms whilst throwing yourself a little backwards. (Fig. 15.)

Fig. 14.

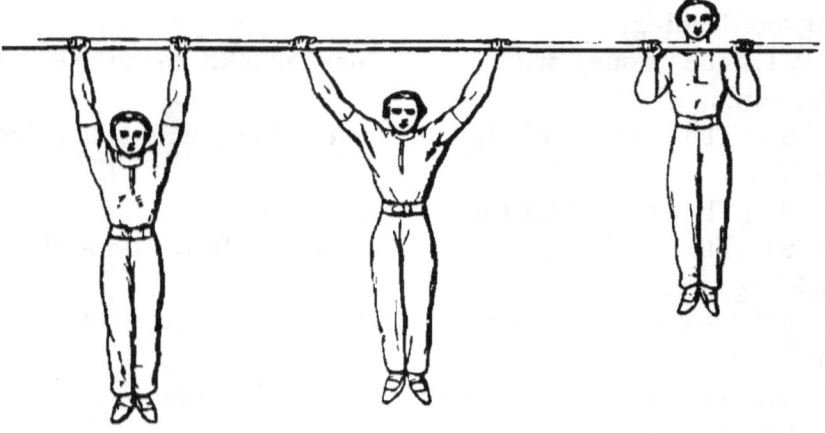

4. With the pole fixed, slowly draw up the feet to the level of the bar, and then let yourself down slowly. (Fig. 16.)

Fig. 15.

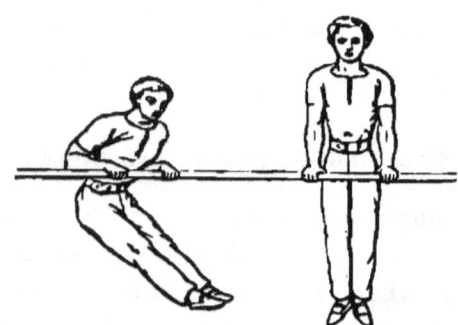

5. Instead of letting yourself down, put the feet slowly between the arms, and then fall to the ground. (Fig. 16.)

6. Instead of passing your feet through the arms carry them steadily over the bar. (Fig. 16.)

7. Swing slowly first, and then boldly whilst hanging on

GYMNASTICS. 87

the bar, until the body can be swung through half a circle, and at length through the whole, or great circle, or entirely round the bar.

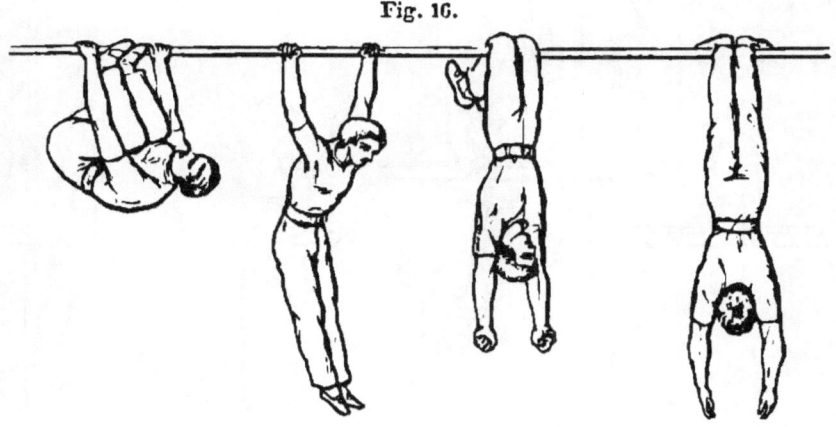

Fig. 16.

8. Whilst hanging on the bar, jump from one end to the other.

9. The trussed fowl and the true lovers' knot are very difficult, and require care lest the wrist should be sprained.

10. *Hanging from the bar by the legs.*—When sitting on the bar quickly slide down backwards perpendicularly, hooking yourself by the legs underneath the knee joint, and having the arms extended in the direction of the body. (Fig. 16.)

11. *Hanging by the feet.*—When the feet are brought to the pole, face the toes upwards, and hitch the insteps over the pole, after which the hands should be loosened and the body allowed to fall perpendicularly without swing or jerk. (Fig. 16.)

TWO PARALLEL BARS.

These bars are about 26 inches apart, and each is fixed at the end upon two strong posts about 4 feet high.

1. Stand between them and take the first position by springing up, and, with the arms quite straight, place a hand on each bar, and remain suspended with the body above the bars. (Fig. 17.)

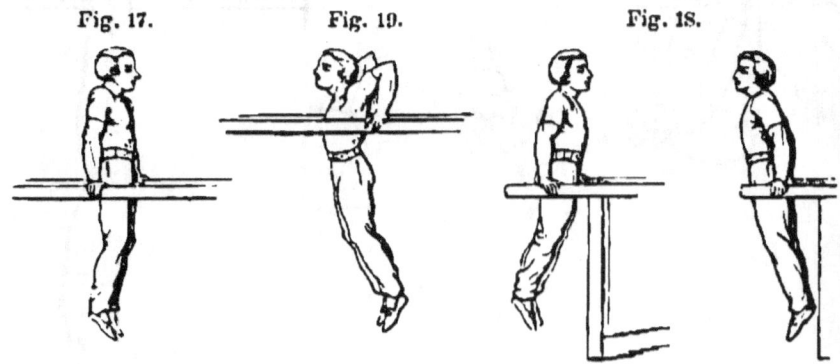

Fig. 17. Fig. 19. Fig. 18.

2. Then walk backwards and forwards, suspended as before. (Fig. 18.)
3. Swing the legs and body backwards and forwards between the bars. (Fig. 20.)

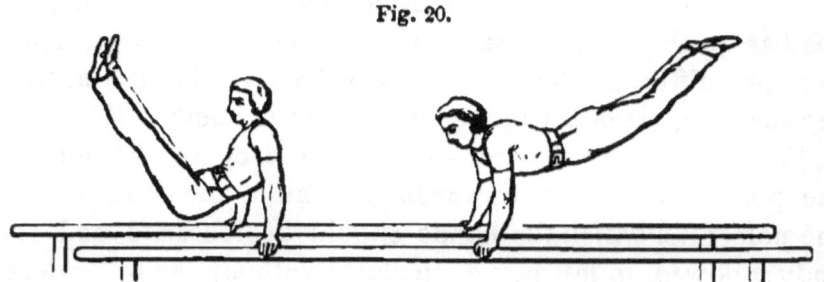

Fig. 20.

4. Draw up the legs at a right angle to the body, and then let the body up and down by straightening and bending the arms.
5. Do the same with the legs pending. (Fig. 19.)

GYMNASTICS. 89

6. With the arms laid along the bars, after taking the first position draw up the body, and swing backwards and forwards.

7. From the first position raise up the legs together and sit upon either bar.

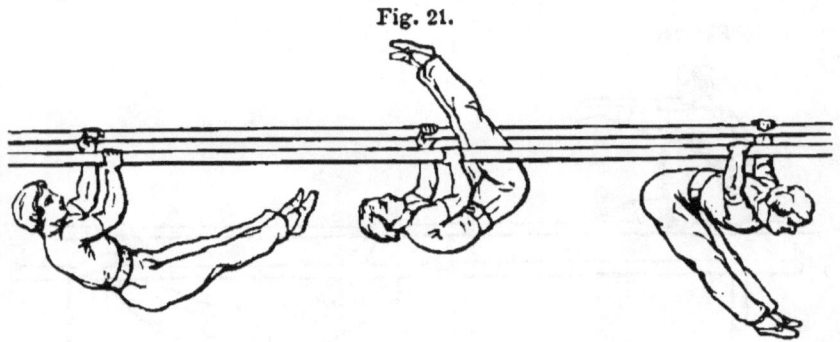

Fig. 21.

8. Spring carefully in the central line so as to throw the whole body from one end to the other, alighting on the bars with the hands. (Fig. 22.)

9. Kneel upon both bars with the hands placed on them,

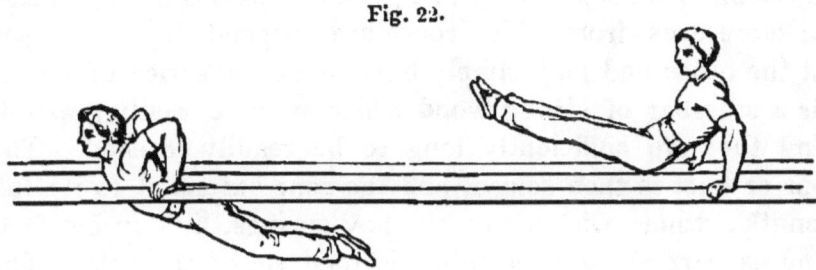

Fig. 22.

and then slide the hands forward and the feet backward, and allow the body to fall so that it will hang by the hands and toes both from the inside of the bars. (Fig. 23.)

10. Sit on one of the bars with one foot hitched under it. (Fig. 24.)

11. Then draw up the other foot and place it on the bar, and by the toe draw yourself upright. (Fig. 24.)

12. With the hands grasping both bars on the outside, draw up the legs carefully, and pass them over the head, hanging by the arms, and then return. (Fig. 21.)

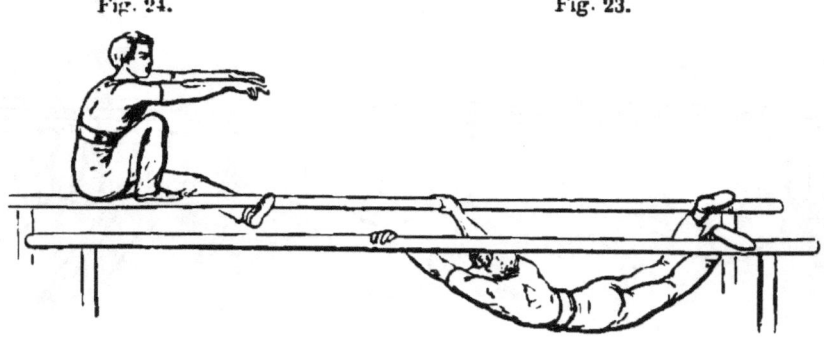

Fig. 24.   Fig. 23.

THE GIANT STRIDE.

An upright and strong pole is fixed firmly into the ground and stands fifteen feet above it. At the top a strong travelling iron cap is fixed in a pivot and passes through three or more eyes, from which ropes are suspended. The ropes at the other end may simply have one or a series of knots, or a crossbar of strong wood which may be easily grasped, and they are sufficiently long to be readily reached. The bar or knot is then seized, and the rope extended to its full length; when, with a run, the boy springs, lifts up his feet, and is carried to a certain distance round the pole. The jump may be repeated or the swing may be kept up by a few touches of the ground with his toes. This should be practised in both directions, and attempts made to jump as high as possible, either without or over a line up to ten feet high.

CLIMBING THE ROPE.

The rope is safely suspended, and should be one inch in thickness. It should be seized firmly by the hands and ascended by extending one hand as much above the other as possible, and descended in the same manner. This will not be possible at first, and the beginner should also seize the rope with his feet, using the foot-hold on the rope as a fulcrum in ascending. (Figs. 25 and 26.)

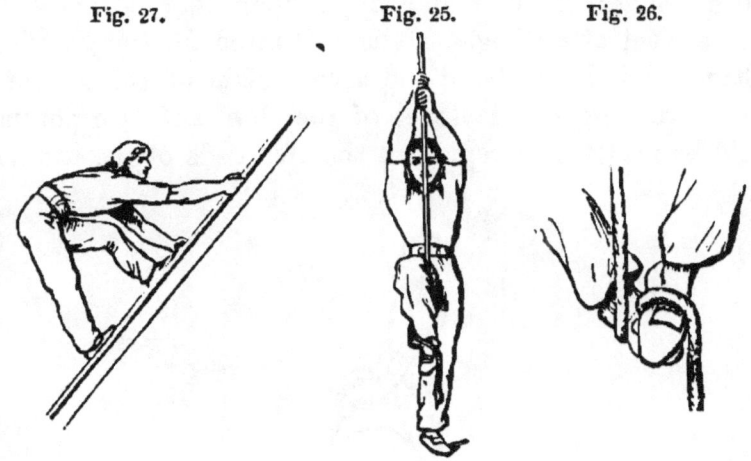

Fig. 27.   Fig. 25.   Fig. 26.

CLIMBING THE POLE.

This scarcely needs description since every boy climbs a tree by grasping it with his arms and legs, and raising them higher alternately. When climbing a palm-tree with very smooth sides, the Indians fix a bandage round both their waist and the tree, and then planting the feet firmly to the trunk, quickly and safely ascend the highest palms.

When the pole is greased it is a difficult task to ascend it by the arms and hands alone, even when the feet are bare.

CLIMBING A BOARD.

The board may be placed at any angle, but at the first lesson it should be tolerably flat. The edges are seized by the fingers, whilst the body is carried up by the advance of the feet in very short steps. (Fig. 27.)

THE WOODEN HORSE.

This may be simply the trunk of a tree about twelve or sixteen inches in diameter fixed upon four straight legs which are set at an angle. It is well fitted for the practice of vaulting, and should be at the usual height of the saddle on a horse, viz., nearly the level of the chin, and two pommels should be inserted to represent the two ends of the saddle.

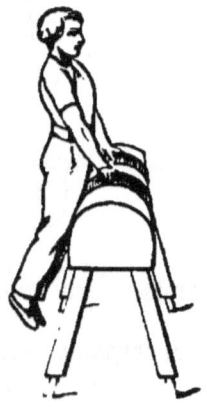

Fig. 28.

1. *To mount.* Seize the pommels and spring up until the straightened arms rest upon the horse (Fig. 28), and then throw the right leg over it. The advantage of this practice is not in the mounting only but in the agility which is gained by springing up from the toes.

In dismounting, first raise the body from the saddle by

placing the hands on the fore pommel of the saddle, and then throw the right leg over and alight on the toes. This may be varied by preventing the toes touching the ground and again vaulting into the saddle. (Fig. 29.)

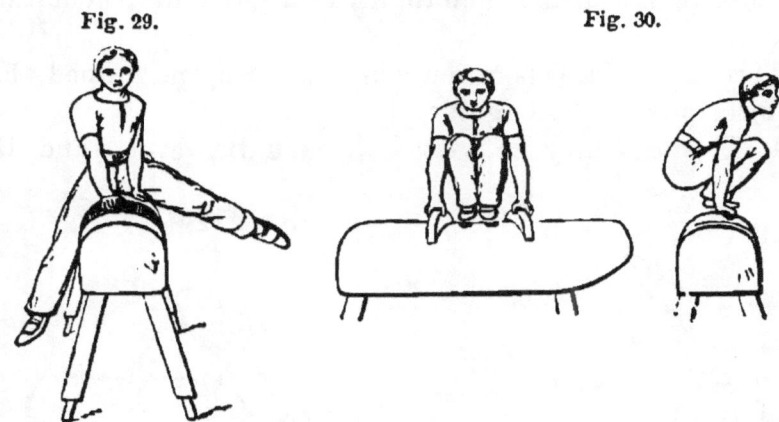

Fig. 29. Fig. 30.

These two series of actions should be repeated in order to gain elasticity and agility.

2. The position of the face may be easily reversed. Mount

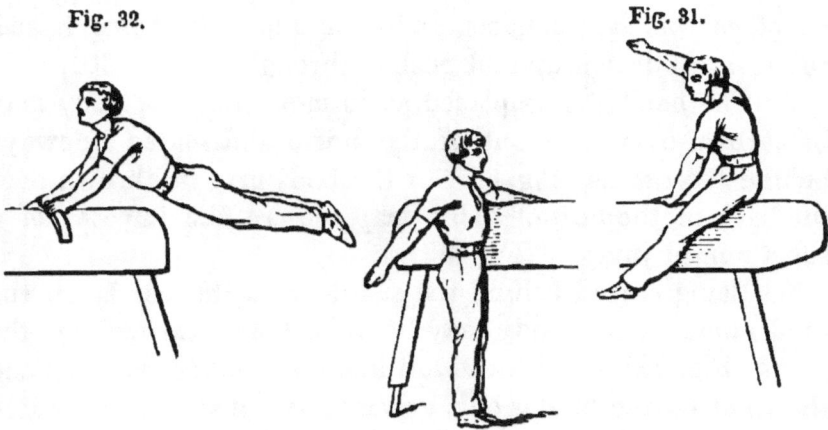

Fig. 32. Fig. 31.

behind the saddle, and then placing the hands on the two

pommels rise up and swing round so as to alight in the saddle. (Figs. 29, 33.)

3. With both hands on the front pommel, swing high in the air with the legs crossed and alight in the saddle with the face reversed, and then return by a swing in the contrary direction.

This is not an operation which is easily performed, but requires practice and agility.

4. The legs may be passed through the arms, and the

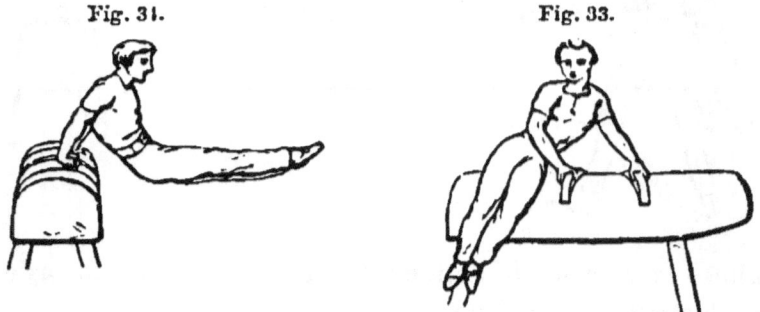

Fig. 31.   Fig. 33.

dismount occur on the off side. This requires the hands to be placed on the pommels, and then the body being raised the feet are drawn up and pushed through. (Fig. 30.)

5. The hands being placed as in mounting, the body may be thrown over the front of the horse and seated sideways behind the saddle (Fig. 33), or the body may be thrown over the back of the horse. This may require the impetus of a short run or jump. (Fig. 32.)

6. Being seated behind the saddle with the hands on the hind pommel, the body may be raised and thrown off the horse (Fig. 32), or with the left hand on the fore pommel and the right on the hinder one, you may swing so as to be seated before the saddle with your face looking backward. (Fig. 33.) The somersault is shown on Fig. 34.

CHAPTER VI.
REST AND SLEEP.

REST.

ALTHOUGH the body is a working machine, and the mind which acts through it is immaterial, they cannot be exercised without intermission, if life is to be maintained. Work and rest are twin sisters, and each must have its sway in turn. "All work and no play, makes Jack a dull boy," has long passed into a proverb, and is an expression of a natural law applicable to all mankind and at all times.

This rest is of two kinds, viz., that which immediately follows fatigue, or a sense of inability to continue to make exertion, and that which is prolonged through a whole day, during a great part of which the body could work. The necessity of the former is apparent, because the mind is conscious of diminished present ability to work; but the latter has not always been allowed, since it is the result of long observation and of reasoning rather than of instinctive conviction.

Experience has shown that men cannot perform laborious work beyond two, three, or four hours at a time without requiring temporary rest; and as this corresponds with the temporary effect of food, the meal-hour has become also the hour of rest. But with the recurrence of each period for work, the sense of fatigue and the necessity for rest become greater, so that at the end of the second period of four hours' work in a day, the body is more fatigued than at the end of the first. The degree varies with many causes, such as the amount of labour required, the capability for labour, and the state of the weather; so that the question of the proper duration of a day's work is not easily answered. Twelve hours has hitherto been regarded as a fair standard, but in many occupations the day is extended to fourteen or sixteen, or contracted to eight or ten hours. Even if the powers of the body were to be taken as the only test, it would not be easy to lay down a universal rule; but the effect of the mind, and the anxieties of life upon the powers of the body must be considered, and the advantage of allowing leisure for the cultivation of the faculties of the mind, as well as for the discharge of the duties of the body, cannot now be overlooked.

One cause of the sense of fatigue is due to the disturbance of the circulation; for one who has walked much finds his feet swollen and his shoes tighter, or if he has used his arms much, finds his hand larger immediately afterwards; but the chief reason is the necessity for the feeding of the muscles, or, as it is termed, the repairing of the waste after labour, since with labour there is much waste and little repair, whilst with rest there is much repair and little waste. Hence we see why it is that the sense of fatigue increases as the day advances, and disappears after the night's rest. This must not be confounded with the receiving of food into the body, for, as will be shown farther on, food thus eaten must be digested before it can nourish, and must be circulated in the muscles before it can repair them. Hence there must be at all times food in the blood in a state fit for use, and the muscles must have intervals of rest, in which they have time, so to speak, to nourish themselves, and to be again strengthened, and ready for a proper period of labour. Hence we see the close connection which exists between the circumstances which, together, make health, viz., labour, food —proper in quantity and quality—good digestion of food, rest for the full use of food, and reinvigoration of the working powers of the body.

The effect of labour upon the circulation begins to be removed when rest commences, so that the sense of fulness of the hands, feet, and head very quickly lessens; but if the exertion has been considerably prolonged, rest is requisite to restore the balance. This is, however, assisted by the posture of the body, as every one knows who after walking raises his legs on a chair, and is soon conscious of the diminished pressure of his boots; but it is rendered perfect when the whole body is laid horizontally. This is explained by the fact that when the body is erect the heart must force the blood upwards to the head, and becomes fatigued; and as the tendency of the blood is to fall in spite of the heart, the circulation is carried on with greater difficulty as the upright position is prolonged. But when the body is horizontal, this difficulty almost vanishes, and the blood is moved along by a smaller propelling force. Moreover, it is a fact, which will be more fully described hereafter, that in this posture of greater ease the circulation is also slower, and the heart is relieved in both ways.

With the short intervals of rest during the day, and the long interval of the night, followed, as they usually are, by so marked a sense of relief, is there any necessity on this ground for any further relaxation? It is an ordinance which has long existed that man should rest one day in seven; and however it may be objected to or abused, it is nominally allowed by all civilised nations, so that every nation has its

Sabbath, although on different days of the week. This has a religious bearing, which should occupy the highest place, as affording leisure for the reception and contemplation of religious truths, and particularly of such as refer to our future state, and for the performance of works of charity and piety, for which time could not be afforded on the other days of the week. But the experience of man has shown that it is perhaps equally important in its bearing upon the fitness of the mind and body to discharge the duties of this life.

If we are conscious of a sense of fatigue with real labour as the day advances, is it not equally true that the sense increases as the week advances, and that whilst the Monday morning finds us fresh and vigorous, and "wound up for the week," on the Friday and Saturday mornings we are much less so; and, in fact, that in any occupation which really taxes the powers of the body, more and better work is done in the early than in the later half of the week. Do we not long for the rest of the Sunday as that day draws nearer and nearer?

But this has been proved to be based upon truth by direct enquiry. In a long series of experiments as to the quantity of food eaten and drank, the amount of waste thrown out of the body, and the weight of the body, I proved that the following changes take place during each week of really hard and regular work:—

1. The appetite gradually lessens, so that less food is eaten at the end than at the beginning of the week.

2. The digestion and use of food is lessened in the same manner, so that there is less waste removed by the kidneys and more by the bowels.

3. The weight of the body is lessened in the same manner at the end of the week.

4. With the rest of the Sunday there is improved appetite

and digestion, so that on the Monday and following days the weight of the body is increased, and the quantity of waste material issuing by the kidneys largely increased also.

The same results have been observed by those who work horses without a day's rest. The horses lose appetite, become thinner, lose spirits, and are dull and sluggish, become less able to work, and at length die earlier. It is now a fixed belief of those who have the care of such animals, that it is cheaper to lose their work one day in the week than to work them every day, and that no increase in quality or quantity of food can obviate the ill-effects of labour continued without intermission.

Do we therefore need further evidence of the wise prohibition of labour on the Sunday for man and animals, and, regarding the subject only in the point of view of health, is not he the wiser who refrains from bodily labour on that day?

The necessity for this rest must vary with the degree of labour of the week, so that the idler may be said not to need that which is of the highest utility to the working man. It is a matter of congratulation that the workers are infinitely more numerous than the drones of society, and if all do not work hard with their bodies, they are not idle in either body or mind. So the degree of rest varies also; for it is not pretended that it is to be absolute, and that no motion should be made on Sunday. A really hard-working man may require more bodily rest than one who makes little exertion. Grahame writes:

"Hail, Sabbath! thee I hail the poor man's day."

Yet a moderate degree of action on the Sunday is necessary to obtain relief for the mind, and to discharge our religious duties, and he who sleeps away the Sunday may as much abuse the day as he who spends it in running hither and thither in pursuit of pleasure. A proper discharge of the special duties of the day, associated with observation of the works of nature, and reflection in country fields and pure air, when such is conveniently practicable, seem to be that which is the most conducive to health of body and mind. Tennyson sings:—

> "On to God's house the people press'd,
> Passing the place where each must rest,
> Each enter'd like a welcome guest."
> * * * * *
> "And forth unto the fields I went,
> And Nature's living motion lent
> The pulse of hope to discontent."

So, in reference to yet longer intervals, the English people of every class have arrived at the conclusion that a respite from daily labour for a few days or weeks in a year, when other scenes may be sought, and present troubles and labour forgotten, is as wise as it is agreeable; and thanks to cheap railway trains and steamboat trips, combined with improved income, this practice will, doubtless, further increase. The meal hours, the night's rest, the Sabbath, and the yearly holiday, are the silken cords which bind the powers of the body together.

SLEEP.

Sleep is necessary to life and health, and the following are its chief effects. The body is at rest by lying down, and unconsciousness; pulsation and respiration are at their lowest point, and allow more rest to the heart and lungs; the circulation is the most easy, for the column of blood is horizontal, and all the actions of the body are at their lowest point. The eyes and ears are at rest by darkness, silence, and unconsciousness. The mind is oblivious, and troubles are forgotten. On awaking, the mind is fresher, the senses acuter, the spirits more cheerful, and all the powers of the body revivified and fitted for work.

Sleep is more or less sound according to circumstances. Fatigue, if not too great, aids it, whilst idleness lessens it. Food, if taken too late, so as not to be digested, and if either too much or too little, lessens it. Some kinds of food, as tea and coffee, may prevent it. Anxious thought and pain, or even great pleasure, lessen it. In proportion as it is sound the body and mind are refreshed.

Hence the conditions most conducive to sleep are previous moderate exertion; light suppers taken at least two hours before going to sleep; no tea or coffee taken at night; calmness of mind and subsidence of thought; a comfortable bed; neither too much nor too little bed-clothing; silence, darkness, moderate warmth and freshness of the air in the bedroom.

Those who work in the night and sleep during the day say that they sleep well; but they have less than those who sleep in the night, and it is much better to sleep in the night than by day.

Sleep is clearly more easily obtained at night during the darkness, and is more difficult when the nights are very short, as at midsummer, than when long, as in mid-winter. With the morning light appearing early, the eyes have not so much rest, and as there is less silence in the streets than in darkness, unconsciousness is less profound and sleep is lighter. Hence there is more and better sleep in winter than in summer.

It is proper to retire to rest early at night, when the day's work is done, and the body and mind are fatigued, and the soundest and best sleep is then obtained. It is said that "one hour's sleep before midnight is better than two afterwards." But when should we awake and get up? Clearly when we are conscious of dreaming, for consciousness has then in great part returned. To awake feeling refreshed, and yet strive to sleep again is to waste time and weaken the body; for every one knows that the second sleep is not so refreshing as the first. Yet many do this, either from sloth or to wait until a fixed hour for rising.

It is difficult to name a given number of hours for sleep at all seasons, but eight hours for an adult, man or woman, and somewhat more for children and old people, is believed to be right. Children naturally sleep long because their bodies need rest for growth, and they go to bed very early; whilst old people are more wakeful, and require to lie down longer than they can sleep.

People generally sleep too much, having regard to their health and the proper use of time, and with the mind at rest a less quantity would be equally good. They should not, however, go to bed late and rise early, but if they must rise early they should go to bed early. Those who go to bed at nine may get up at four or five o'clock, and those who stay up until ten or eleven may rest until five, six, or seven o'clock, according to their age, health, and duties.

The proper rule is to go to bed early and rise early, and to make the best use of the morning hours for devotion and study.

There can be no doubt that to lie down an undue length of time, and to use too much clothing, is to relax the body and to make it less fit for exertion, so that, independently of waste of time, less tone and health of body result. The heart becomes feeble and the skin unusually sensitive, whilst at the same time the lowest state of vital action is unduly prolonged, so that disease, having the character of debility and a tendency to take colds, must follow. On the other hand, to rise when we have been sufficiently refreshed is to add to the usefulness of the body as an instrument of labour and to prolong life. Two hours a day saved from prolonged sleep adds thirty days to every year of life, and every twelve years we shall have practically lived one year longer. We forget this as life passes, but how will it appear when life is ending! The greatest men of all ages have been early risers, so as to find time for their work, and if the young would strive to emulate them they must not waste time, whether in bed or otherwise. Oh! for a single day! is the thought of many at the last; and even those who have spent their time the most usefully feel that there is still much more that they might have done.

CHAPTER VII.

CLEANLINESS AND BATHING.

Cleanliness of the body has at least three advantages: it promotes health, improves the personal appearance, and removes causes of offence to others. So important is it that a great practical divine said that cleanliness is next to godliness. Although cleanliness is not so universal as it should be, it is now much more common than formerly, and a dirty person is not regarded as respectable. No lesson is more important for the young than to learn the necessity for perfect cleanliness of the body; and although they may not be able to accomplish it in its fullest sense, they should make every effort to do so.

When the skin is dirty the pores are covered, and the perspiration which goes on without being noticed, is hindered. This is more important than is generally understood, for it is by means of that kind of perspiration that the body is kept cool, and the heat regulated. In this sense dirt will be more hurtful in summer than in winter, because the cooling of the body is then more needed, but it is required at every hour of the day, and particularly within three hours after meals. It is also more needful in those who have enough to eat than in those who starve. (See Fig. 20, p. 134.)

But besides cooling the body, the skin throws out matters which the body does not need and must get rid of, many of which have a strong odour when allowed to remain on the skin, so that dirty persons smell sour or are otherwise offensive. If not removed from the skin they prevent more from escaping, and the body is obliged to retain that which for health it ought to lose. Further, perspiration with dirt adhering to the skin, which may not be offensive at first, becomes so after a time, and makes the person disagreeable to all about him.

It must not be forgotten that those who have dirty and offensive skins become accustomed to the smell, and do not notice that it is offensive, and thus they are disagreeable and disliked by others, without knowing the cause. This is particularly undesirable, and, when known, is extremely humiliating.

These remarks apply to the whole skin, for every part of it perspires; but more particularly to certain parts. Thus, the face, neck, and hands being uncovered, cool the body more than the parts which are covered, and therefore should be kept particularly clean. The arm-pits and feet give a peculiarly offensive smell, which is perceived through any amount of clothing, and particularly when the person is warm; and therefore should be kept very clean. When woollen shirts are worn next the skin, and particularly in hot weather, and are not changed frequently, and the skin is not cleansed daily, the part of the body which is covered becomes offensive.

In hot weather the perspiration now referred to, and which is called insensible because we do not see it, is greatly increased, and covers the whole body with vapour or fluid. It is partially absorbed by the clothing, but the parts unclad show the drops or streams of water. This is absolutely necessary in those who make much exertion, and if it were possible to stop it, the person must die. Many of those who work hard become very dirty with the dust, as is particularly the case with colliers, or chimney sweeps; and if they are not cleanly, it is most difficult for them to keep in health. Many more diseases are due to want of cleanliness than dirty people are aware of.

From all this, it follows that whilst the hands and face should be cleansed several times a day, the whole body, including the feet, should be washed so frequently as to keep it clean. There is difficulty in many small houses in obtaining conveniences to wash the body all over, but every one may wash below the head, face, and neck, and the feet daily, and when engaged in dirty work, may wash down to the loins. There are now public baths in all the larger towns, and everybody should wash in such a bath once a week, or as often as may be possible.

The use of soap is necessary, and particularly to workmen, and hot water should be used whenever the skin is very dirty. The washing and subsequent rubbing should be thorough, so as to completely cleanse the skin and remove the water. Those who do not make much exertion, and who wash the body daily, find that very little soap and effort are necessary, whilst the ease of washing and sense of comfort are very great. Try to do this, and you will find it become easier and more agreeable every day.

The use of clean clothing is nearly as important as washing the skin, for a clean skin and a dirty, sour-smelling shirt do not agree. So also a person cannot be called clean who wears dirty outer clothes, whether gowns or coats, however clean the skin may be; but, in fact, a person who willingly wears dirty clothes does not well wash the skin. Cleanliness of skin will cause cleanliness everywhere, and is one of the best motives for tidiness. For the same reason, a person who has a clean skin will not wilfully cause unnecessary dirt in anything or anywhere, and therefore becomes a more agreeable neighbour.

Those who handle substances which may cause disease have far greater reasons for cleanliness than others, and such are plumbers and chimney-sweeps. If they would wash their skin frequently, the dangerous matter would not be absorbed into the blood, and they would be spared from colic, skin disease, and cancer. It is carelessness on this subject that has produced permanent palsy of the wrist and hand in many a water-gilder, and liability to lead poisoning in plumbers and painters. In every occupation lay down the fundamental rule that you will not injure your health for want of a little soap and water.

Bathing is, no doubt, a part of washing and cleanliness, for one cannot bathe in clean water without becoming cleaner, but it is used for health on other grounds.

Cold baths when properly taken, harden the skin and make it less liable to take colds, and must therefore be useful. It is, however, necessary to use reasonable caution. As the water is colder than the body it may take away too much heat suddenly, which would weaken, and might even bring on cramp which has caused many to be drowned. It is, therefore, desirable not to stay too long in the water, and to keep moving when in it, and probably five minutes is as long as the bath should be continued. Some remain in so long that they are very cold and exhausted and feel worse for bathing, whilst others remain in for a long time in order to learn to swim ; and as everybody should learn that art they may be excused, if they suffer no perceptible harm. In all such cases the skin should be well rubbed afterwards, so as to produce a glow of heat, and if very cold, a cup of hot coffee with hot milk should be drunk, whilst in extreme cases the person should go to bed and be covered with blankets or be put into a hot bath.

When a cold slipper-bath is taken the water should not be too cold, and as no exertion can be made it should not be continued more than two or three minutes. Cold bathing in a house should, however, be restricted to plunging, sponging, and shower-baths, which are over in a very short time. In warm weather nothing is more beneficial or more easily accomplished than a shower-bath, and the cost of the apparatus is now very small.

Sea bathing is the best mode of cold bathing, since the waves compel the bather to move about, and the salt prevents colds; but, even then, the duration of the bath should not exceed five minutes. It is important to cover the whole body with water, so that all parts may be equally cold, and perhaps nothing more is required than to duck over head a few times and then go out. Much of the present bathing of women and children in the sea is useless, if not something worse.

Sea bathing is usually taken as an amusement by persons in health, with pleasure and impunity, but it is very different with those who are in a state of disease. With the water at 55° and the body at 98° it is clear that the latter will very speedily lose much heat, and if the appetite for food, or the digestion of food, be insufficient, it may be very injurious. Consumptive and very feeble people should take such baths with the greatest caution, and under medical advice. On the other hand operatives, who become dirty in the performance of their duties, may thus cleanse the skin, but less easily than in fresh water.

The portion of salt which remains upon the skin is very valuable in stimulating that organ and preventing colds.

CHAPTER VIII.

CONDITION OF DWELLINGS.

HOUSES.

Houses should be roomy, dry, light, and well ventilated, situated in a healthful locality, and surrounded by everything conducive to health. How far is the actual state of houses from this description; and how impossible is it for the poor, and in some places for any class, to obtain a proper residence! Yet we will assume that if more knowledge on this subject existed among tenants an improved state of things would be provided by landlords, and will describe that which should be sought for.

The site of a house should be high and dry. High, in order that the winds may blow upon it from all quarters and the air about it be less damp than in the valleys. It is well known that in winter the site of a house on a hill is less cold than one lying low in a neighbouring valley, for whilst vegetation may be uninjured in the former it may be frost-bitten in the latter. This is due chiefly to the air being more damp in the latter than in the former. It should be dry, so that foul water may not remain about the house, and that moderate drainage may suffice to carry off all rain and other water. This is partly due to the character of the soil, but chiefly to the perfection of the drainage. If the soil be sandy it will absorb foul slops and other water, and so appear dry on the surface, whilst at a depth of a few inches it may hold a great quantity of water which no drainage could entirely remove. Do not therefore be deceived by the appearance of the surface, but see that the ground is kept dry by drains.

A clay soil is cold unless it be well drained, for the water lies upon it and makes the air damp, and the sun's heat does not warm it. Undrained clay must be injurious to health, but well-drained clay need not do harm.

Grass land around a house is cooler in summer and warmer in winter than arable land.

The surface should be well drained by surface-drains, because of the rains and slops, and the gutters should be laid so as to carry off the water perfectly, and be kept clean. They should lead into underground drains, or carry the water entirely off the premises. No surface or underground drain should go near a well, and no slops or dirt should be thrown near a well, lest the water should be fouled. The underground drains are not readily seen, but they should be known to the tenant. Many are ill-made of broken bricks, and allow the foul water to stand in them, or to run through their sides. They should be made of glazed earthenware pipes, soundly joined together.

Where there are grates leading into such drains, there should be traps which will prevent the foul air coming back into the house or premises, and this is particularly necessary when the drains lead into a pit or cesspool, which is closed over, and does not otherwise allow the foul gases to escape. Wherever there are cesspools they should be ventilated by stand-pipes, so that foul air cannot accumulate; and where there are sewer drains inside a house or yard, they should be ventilated in the same manner.

In the country the petty should be kept very clean, the pit covered with ashes, and there should be a roof to keep out the rain. If there is any overflow from it, see that it does not go near the well, and have it cleared away constantly. It is better to have earth or ash-closets which do not need any pits. They are simply boxes placed under the seat, and dry earth or ash is thrown in after the petty is used. When the box is full it is carried out and emptied into the garden, and the contents used as manure. The simplicity and efficiency of the plan are very great.

In towns where there are water-closets see that the apparatus is in good repair, and that there is plenty of water, and take care that nothing be thrown down that might stop up the closet. Do not draw water for drinking from a cistern which supplies a closet. If you perceive a foul smell from the closet, sink, or grating, be sure that there is something wrong, and that you may have fever unless it be put right.

If there be a pigsty do not have it very near the house. Keep it very clean, and do not allow manure to accumulate, but carry it away and cover it with earth until it is ready for use on the land. Be careful that there is no filthy water running from the sty, or manure, or any that can go near the well.

Do not leave heaps of filth or rubbish near the house, and be sure to keep the surface of the ground well washed, clean, and dry.

The well should not be very near the house, petty, or pigstye, and should be covered over, and the top should be higher than the ground. Be watchful if there should be any doubt on these things.

WARMTH.

Houses should be kept reasonably warm, which implies means of cooling in summer, and of heating in winter.

Sufficient care is not taken in this country to protect our rooms from the full influence of the sun in summer, so that some of the bedrooms are insufferably hot when entered at night, and really unfit for habitation, whilst the heat of the living rooms causes profuse perspiration, which is not of an agreeable odour, and tends to excite decomposition in food or other articles. We rarely provide any other protection than a white calico blind, and, if shutters are attached to the windows, they are rarely closed for this purpose. Outside venetian shutters are as uncommon here as they are universal in France and Italy; but they have the advantage of excluding the hottest rays of the sun, whilst they admit a current of air, and are most valuable. The inside venetians are more frequently used than formerly, and are desirable, but are altogether inferior to the outside shutters, both in excluding the sun and admitting air. Whilst warmth is healthful, too much heat causes relaxation, and particularly in children, so that a very hot room is almost always disagreeable and unhealthful. A south-west aspect is better for this purpose than a southern one, since the full power of the sun is exerted upon the front of the house for a shorter period, and where there is (as there should always be) a front and back, one part of the house may be cool when the other is hot. It is also desirable that there should be protection afforded by trees, so that some part of the immediate neighbourhood may have shade, and afford a cool retreat; but they should not entirely surround the house, or be very near it, lest they should induce damp.

The warming of houses is still in a very rude state in this

country. The first plan is seen in barbarous nations of having a fire in the middle of the room, and an opening in the roof for the exit of the smoke. The next step was to convert the hole into a tube by building a chimney, and to remove the fireplace to the side wall, and then we had a hearth with or without "dogs," on which the fuel was burnt, a wide, open hearth place, higher than a man, and a chimney leading to the roof. The third stage is that which is now almost universal—that is to say, the hearth-place is filled below with a fire grate, intended for heating and cooking, and above by bricks and stone, so that the chimney is brought down quite, or nearly to the grate.

With this arrangement the heat is given out on one side of a room, and cannot therefore warm each part equally, and the larger proportion goes up the chimney, and is lost.

What is required is a system by which all the heat shall be saved, and distributed where it is required.

When a stove is placed in the middle of the room, as in France and Germany, the heat is more uniformly distributed to all parts; and as a pipe is attached to it which conveys the heated smoke and air, and passes through the room, it also distributes heat, and saves much of that which now passes up the chimney. It is not too much to affirm that, by such an arrangement, the room would be better warmed with one-third of the quantity of fuel now used with the ordinary grate and chimney. Moreover, the pipe, or flue, from such a stove, could be made to pass through the hall or bedrooms, and thus warm them without any increase of cost, and keep rooms dry, which, being but little used, are liable to be damp. Such stoves are made with various degrees of ornament, and at prices within the reach of all classes, and, if encased in earthenware, are not liable to burn objects touching them.

Rooms may be equally well warmed without either stove

or fire-grate, by carrying around them a flue from a stove, or pipes circulating hot water from a boiler in the kitchen or elsewhere. This would probably be the most economical mode of warming rooms if the houses were adapted to it when constructed, and the trouble and expense of keeping them in order is very small. Moreover, the heat thus distributed may be regulated, and the supply cut off at any moment.

The pleasure afforded by an open fire in our rooms has hitherto hindered the general adoption of these plans, for abundance of coal has not made it too costly; but it is merely a sentiment, and, in its absence, we should soon find that social pleasure depends much more upon ourselves than upon a bright and cheerful-looking fire.

It is scarcely practicable to fix upon a temperature which should be maintained at all seasons, for that which would feel warm in winter would be cold in summer. Perhaps 54° to 60° in winter, and 60° to 64° in summer, is the most agreeable temperature.

When coal is used, the chief inconvenience is the dirt and dust which it occasions, whether in bringing it into the room, in its combustion, or in cleaning the grate, and these cost no little in labour, brushes, and furniture. When charcoal is used, there is the danger of suffocation by carbonic acid gas, which it produces in burning, and, if allowed to escape in the room, will render the air unwholesome. Many persons have been found dead in bedrooms which were closed, when there was a charcoal fire. With such fuel there should be perfect means of removing the heated air, and the rooms should not be closed. If the air should feel heavy and oppressive, and cause an inclination to sleep, the windows and doors should be opened, and the foul air allowed to escape.

It is, however, more common in this country to burn charcoal in stoves in workshops than in dwelling rooms, and the irritating fumes which are thus inhaled cause irritation of the throat of the most troublesome kind, and chronic cough. Whenever such fumes are perceived, the charcoal should be discontinued.

Gas is also used both to give heat and light, and produces fumes of a sulphurous and irritating nature. Diseases of the eyes and nose, and bronchitis are much more commonly due to this cause than is generally allowed, and the more so that no special means are provided for the removal of the fumes. Whenever the smell is offensive or irritating, it indicates that better ventilation is required, as no one should willingly breathe air thus made impure.

The supply of gas also causes explosions and suffocation when it escapes from the pipes into a room. Gas by itself does not explode, but when it is mixed with the air, and a light is introduced, it may do so with the most serious consequences. Whenever therefore there is a smell of gas, the windows and doors should be opened, and no fire or light admitted until it has been removed.

There is no danger of explosion in the small amount which escapes without causing a smell of gas, but it is often injurious to health, and causes headache, lowness of spirits, and loss of appetite. In this minute quantity it rather resembles a sewer smell than that of gas. When the quantity is considerable it may cause suffocation, and many deaths have been due to it.

Hence the use of gas is attended with no little injury to health, and with some risk of explosion, and the utmost care should be taken that the pipes and joints should be perfect, the taps turned, and the supply cut off at the meter when the gas is not required. There should also be proper means of ventilation. A small fishtail gas-burner consumes as much air as a man.

When a chimney is on fire, the opening at the bottom should be entirely and quickly stopped up, so as to prevent any air being admitted into it.

The use of petroleum for giving light and heat is often attended by danger of explosion or of fire, since it burns at a temperature far below that of boiling water. If allowed to escape, and then ignited, it may burn the house down, and therefore the utmost care should be taken to prevent this. It should be obtained in small quantities at a time, be kept in well-corked tin cans in a cool place, and never poured out in a room with a fire or a light. It is dangerous to burn it in glass fountains, lest the lamp should be thrown down, and the glass should break. Silber's lamps are good, inasmuch as they are of metal, and only a few drops of the petroleum can be burnt at a time.

VENTILATION.

An ill-ventilated house is almost sure to bring fever, and a house to be well ventilated must have in every room means for the air to come in and go out.

Houses built back to back cannot be well ventilated, and should not be inhabited. All houses should have windows and doors at the front and back, which should be opened every day, so that a draught may go through them.

The windows should be made to open, and should be opened as the weather will allow.

The living rooms may be well ventilated when the bedrooms are ill ventilated, for the doors are very frequently opened, and people go in and out; whilst the doors and windows of the bedrooms are kept shut. Therefore pay particular attention to the ventilation of the bedroom, and see that there are two openings into it through which air may pass all the night. The chimney of the bedroom is often stopped up to prevent the dust and soot falling, but as this prevents ventilation it is very improper. Better to have dust, which can be cleared away, than bad health and fever.

It is often very difficult to ventilate a bedroom without giving colds, because no one should sleep in a draught, and disease is sometimes produced by thoughtlessly having too much ventilation. If the door be left a very little open by using a peg or chain, and a window be opened at the top for half an inch, it will usually be enough to secure moderate ventilation, and the bed should be placed out of the draught; but the amount must be tested by the smell of the room, and if in the morning it is disagreeable, it will be necessary to have more ventilation.

Neither put the bed in a draught nor in a corner so far away that the air about it cannot be purified by ventilation, and take care that there is bedclothing proportionate to the ventilation. Never let the bedroom, or any room, become too warm for want of ventilation, and then open a door or window to cool it, for by so doing you will be sure to give colds; but keep a proper temperature from the beginning. Take care also that the rooms are not too cold by ventilation, or you may greatly injure the health of children and old people, but let everything be done with judgment and moderation.

If there are no means of ventilation besides the door, window, and chimney, and the doors and windows fit closely, you should have ventilating bricks of the size of an ordinary brick put into the walls close to the ceiling, and if there is a draught from them cover them on the inside with finely perforated zinc.

It is clear that the necessity for ventilation varies very much. Thus, if the house be built on a hill where the winds blow on all sides; the doors and windows, and perhaps the roof allow air to enter freely; if people constantly go in and out; if not too many live in the house, and the weather be cold, there will be less necessity than under the contrary conditions. The two next important questions are the mode of construction of the house, and the number of people in a given space. If the house be overcrowded it cannot be sufficiently ventilated, and this is the case with very many houses of the working men. It is difficult to say what space should be allowed to each person, but in public lodging-houses it is two hundred and forty cubic feet, and two children might be reckoned as one adult.

In all these matters the smell is a good test, for if it be foul, the air is certainly bad, and the house is over-crowded or ill-ventilated, and fewer people or more air is required.

Do not forget that furniture and heaps of rubbish in the house and cupboards fill up space and retain foul air. Keep no old rags or bones, or any other rubbish, in the house, and put away all the clothes into drawers, so that there shall be the least possible hindrance to the circulation of air.

Let special care be taken that the cellar, pantry, and passages are kept sweet and airy, and that no foul smells or rubbish are in them. If they are foul, they will taint the air of the house and the food, and may produce disease.

The rooms, and particularly any that are foul, should be whitewashed every few months, so as to become sweet. Many persons care nothing about the state of those which are not usually seen, but as one room affects another, all are really important for health.

Do not keep heaps of dirty clothes or dirty linen, and particularly the linen used by sick persons, but have them washed as soon as possible. The linen of fever patients should be at once put into a boiler and boiled for half an hour; and no very dirty linen can be well washed if it be not well boiled.

With all this, it is needless to say that the house should be kept perfectly clean by washing and scouring, but if there are boarded floors, do not use dirty water, or too much water, or allow it to drip between the boards. A badly-washed boarded floor is often very offensive to the smell. So also when brick or tile floors are washed, they should be well dried, and the children should not get their feet wet by them.

The roof should be in good order, and neither the floor nor the walls damp. A damp house is almost always unhealthy, and needs better ventilation. If the walls rising from the ground are damp, it may be costly to cure them, but the dampness of floors may be more readily remedied by drainage.

When houses are properly built, dampness is prevented by a damp course, layers of concrete, and drains. Consumption, rheumatism, low fever, and general ill-health, are frequently found in damp houses, and if the damp be incurable, the tenant should leave it. Perhaps there is no one defect in the small houses of the labouring classes so prejudicial to health as damp, if it be at all general.

CHAPTER IX.

SKETCH OF PHYSIOLOGY.

Our bodies are made for exertion, as is shown by the use of the bones and flesh, or, as the latter is called, muscles, so that we can walk and run with our legs, lift and fight with our arms, and carry burdens on our shoulders, and by those agents perform the duties by which men generally gain their living.

But the bones and muscles as they are used, wear away, and need constant repair; and for that purpose food is required. Hence, we must have teeth to chew, palates to taste, throats to swallow, stomachs to digest, and other organs to prepare the food for its use in the body. Besides these, we need the bowels to carry away needless and refuse food, and other organs to get rid of the wasted part of muscles, bones, &c., and some portions of food which are waste, and no longer useful in the body.

All these are of no value in themselves, but necessary to make the body a working machine; and at the same time a good Providence has so arranged that they give us much gratification.

No man can live altogether for work, for he would directly waste away; and no man should live altogether, or chiefly, for eating, or he would be useless to others; but we must eat and work together, and in due moderation.

Further, the body is warm, and in that state is the most fitted for both work and pleasure; and (what is not a little surprising) it is almost equally warm under all circumstances. Here, then, we have a great problem—how to warm the body and to keep it always equally warm.

Besides all this, the body, as a machine or instrument for work, must be guided by intelligence, just as a steam-engine must have an engine-driver; for a muscle or a bone cannot guide and direct itself. Hence we require the mind —the intelligence, by which we know what we desire, and the will, to order the muscles to move. This is done without our perception, and yet we know that we direct it by our mind and will.

Those functions in the body which are needful to maintain life, as the digestion of food, the circulation of the blood, and the breathing of air, go on without our will, and are therefore called *involuntary;* for if they required our will they would stop when we slept, and we should die.

See, then, the beautiful arrangement of Providence:—

We have muscles to enable us to work, and we can direct them by our intelligence and will;

We have organs which repair them, and act without our perception and will, and maintain life either with or without our knowledge and consent;

We have minds which direct and control our bodies and wills, which make us free agents in their use;

We keep the body warm, and at about the same heat at all times, with very little voluntary attention and control;

We get rid of unnecessary and refuse food and wasted muscles and bones, with very little attention and control;

And in all these actions we have so much pleasure that the poor and the rich may enjoy life in not very different degrees.

We will now in a very few words show how these operations take place.

We select food partly by our taste, partly by our experience, and partly by our opportunities and pecuniary means, and in quantities which we find by experience to be necessary, or if more than necessary, such that the body can receive without immediate injury.

The food is almost always a mixture of different things, for nobody willingly makes a meal of one kind of food alone. It is taken in proper portions into the mouth, where it is mixed with a large quantity of saliva, and chewed by the teeth until it is made into a soft, half-fluid mass, when it is swallowed. The amount of chewing required differs very much according to the kind of food, as we know when chewing a piece of tough meat and a well-cooked potato; but it should still be perfectly done. The quantity of the saliva, and the necessity for it, varies; it is the most with bread and all foods containing starch, for by it the starch is changed into sugar. All such foods should be well mixed with it, and not hastily swallowed, or they will not be well digested.

If the food be not soft enough it is sometimes arrested in the throat, and a large piece of meat may stop the breathing, or when it goes lower down it calls upon us to drink water to wash it through the gullet into the stomach.

Having entered the stomach, the digestion of animal food begins, and that of vegetable food is continued. The secretions of the stomach, called the gastric juice, are poured out in large quantity and dissolve the food. The food as it is changed is absorbed into, or drank by certain small vessels, which after a time pour it into the blood-vessels, through which it is conveyed to the heart, and the heart by its beats sends it to all parts of the body. Some of it remains in the

SKETCH OF PHYSIOLOGY. 123

blood, and goes round and round the circulation, but another part stops in the muscles and repairs them. The used part of the muscles and the food which is not wanted is then carried to the kidneys, and is thrown out of the body.

The five following illustrations are intended to show the chief structures connected with the circulation of the blood, and should be examined and studied with care.

The heart is composed of two halves (right and left), but they are not separated as shown in Fig. 35, and each half is

SECTION OF THE HEART.

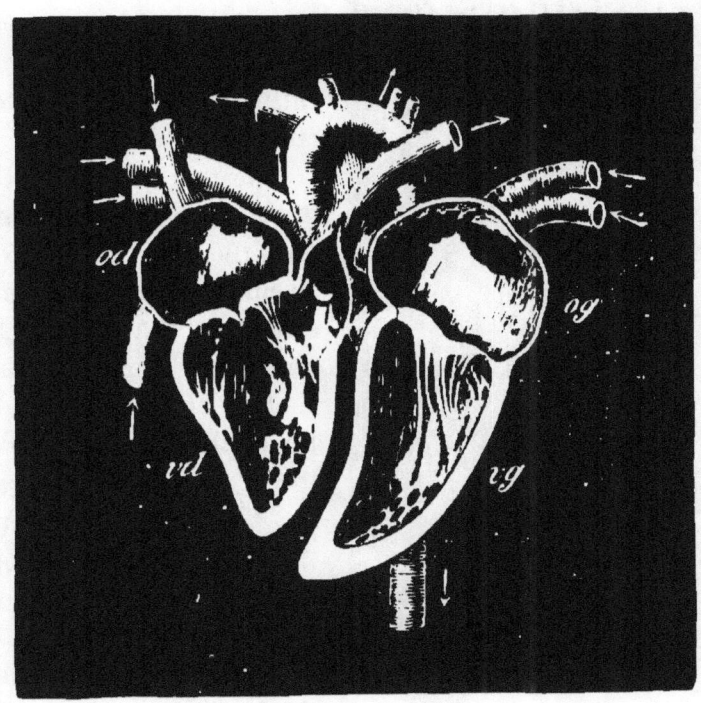

Fig 35.

subdivided. The upper part of each half is called the auricle, and the lower the ventricle. The blood is brought from all

SCHEME OF THE CIRCULATION.

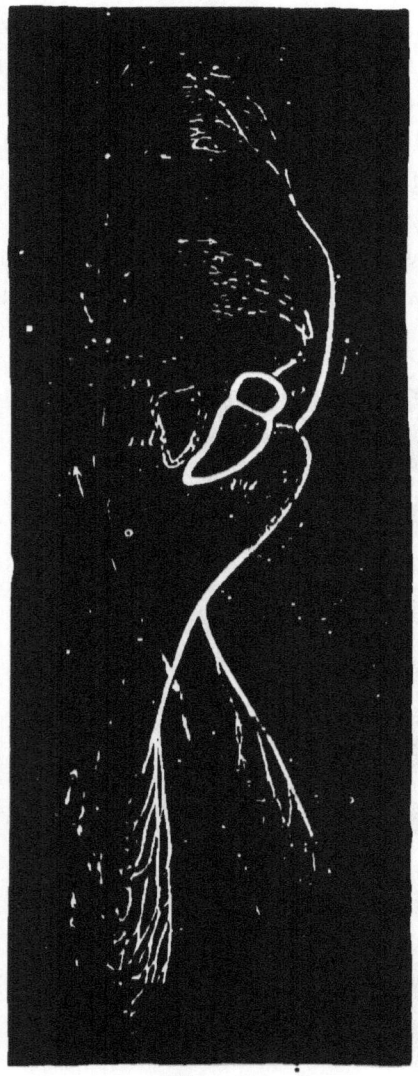

Fig. 36.

parts of the body by the veins to the right auricle, *od*, whence it passes down into the right ventricle, *rd*, and is sent by the pulmonary artery to the lungs. It is brought back from the lungs to the left auricle, *og*, whence it passes to the left ventricle, *rg*, and is sent to all parts of the body.—The direction of the arrows should be noticed, as indicating the course of the circulation.

The two sides of the heart are again shown in Fig. 36, with the great division of the circulation. The uppermost circuit is that to the head, neck, and arms, the middle that of the lungs, and the lower that of the trunk and lower limbs. The lines on the left side of the heart indicate arteries by which the blood is carried from the heart, and on the left, veins by which it is returned to the heart.

The arteries end, and the veins begin in an infinite number of small vessels called capillaries (because they are as fine as a hair), and it is there that the chief chemical actions take place. When magnified they are beautiful and interesting objects, since the circulation and the contents of the vessels are seen, as in Fig. 37, taken from a frog's foot. The capillaries are of different sizes, and branch in various directions, whilst the mass of round or oval bodies within them are the blood corpuscles.

CIRCULATION IN THE FROG'S FOOT.

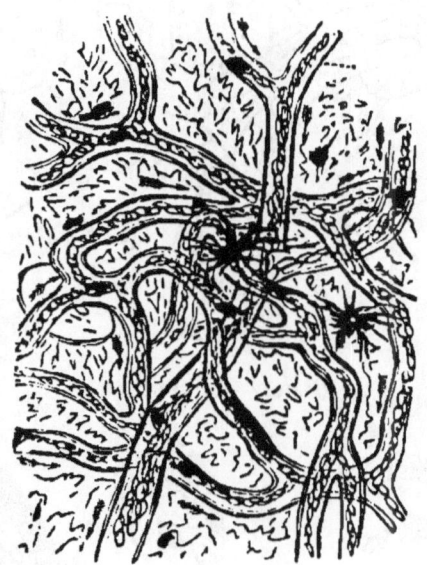

Fig. 37.

A very similar arrangement is found in vegetables, for they, like animals, have a circulation, as may be readily seen in a water-plant called Vallisneria, and in the india-rubber-tree. (Fig. 38.)

The following are the blood corpuscles found in various classes of animals (Fig. 39):—

A, Of man—*a*, red ; *b*, white.
B, Of the pigeon.

C, Of the ray fish—*a* red; *b*, white.
D, Of the proteus.
E, Of insects and molluscs.

CIRCULATION IN THE INDIA-RUBBER PLANT.

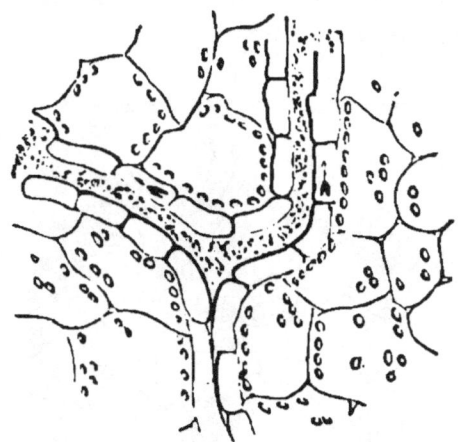

Fig. 38.

BLOOD CORPUSCLES.

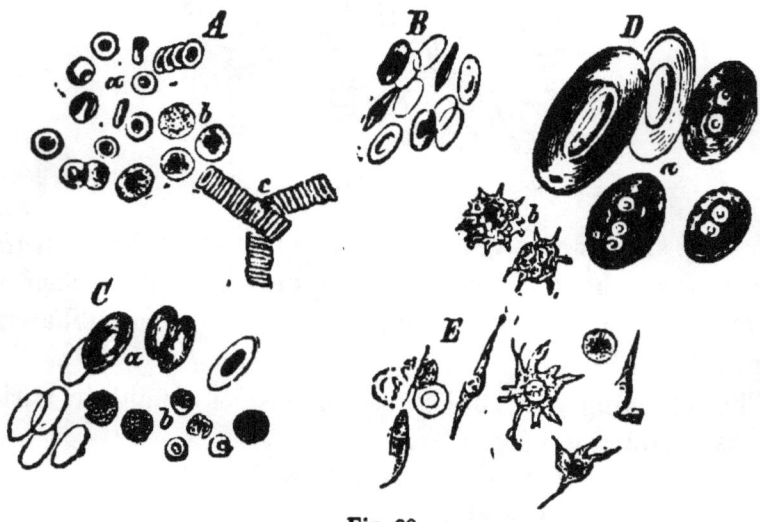

Fig. 39.

These corpuscles circulate in the blood, and as the red ones carry the oxygen of the air, they are redder in arterial than in venous blood. Their different size and form enable us to distinguish the blood of each of the great classes of animals, but not the blood of man, from that of other mammalia, as the ox.

When the food is thus thrown into the blood, and the blood carried to the heart, it is first sent to the lungs, where it meets with the air which has been drawn into them by breathing. It takes up and uses some of this air (oxygen), and gives off gas (carbonic acid) which is made both from it and the used food. The first is carried round the circulation, and the second is thrown out by the lungs, and makes the air so impure that it should not be breathed again.

The Lungs.

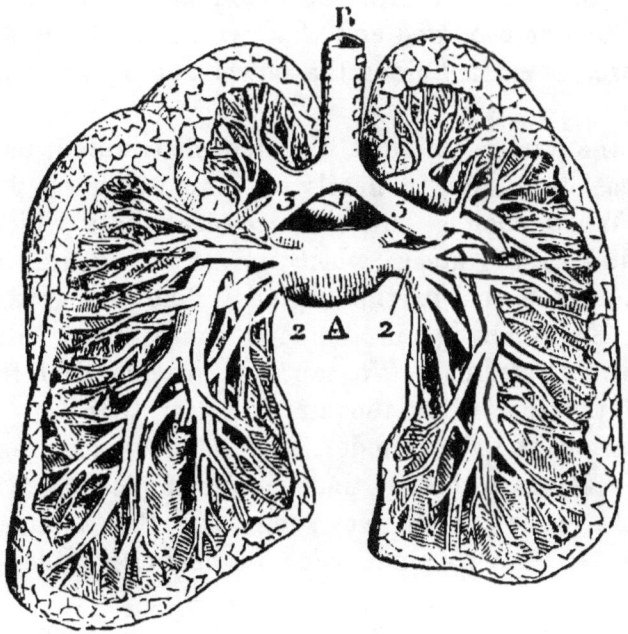

Fig. 40.

In Fig. 40 the lungs have been dissected to show the distribution of the windpipe and bronchi, and the blood vessels; but their usual appearance is shown by the mottled border.

B is the windpipe, dividing into the two bronchi, 3, which go on subdividing until the tube is scarcely larger than a thick pin.

A is the blood vessels which accompany the bronchi.

1 is the pulmonary artery, carrying the blood to the lungs; and 2, the pulmonary veins, carrying it back to the heart.

That part of the food which was not digested in the stomach, or, if digested, was not absorbed into the vessels, is carried into the bowels; and there the fat meets with secretions called the pancreatic juice, and the bile, by which it is dissolved and digested, and with the other digested food is then carried into the blood and proceeds to the heart. The refuse food and that which is still undigested and unused is carried along the bowel and is thrown out of the body.

Thus the food is obtained, digested, distributed, used, and finally cast out; and in nearly all these actions it produces heat. When coal is burnt it produces heat which boils water, and causes steam which moves the steam-engine to work; and the coal in the engine is like the food in our bodies. Every change in the food causes heat within our bodies and warms us. We can also receive heat from the fire and the sun, when the air is hotter than our bodies; but generally the air is colder, and therefore takes heat from us. We regulate this by the amount of clothing which we wear, the fires which we keep, and the shelter which we seek, so that we endeavour to be neither too cold nor too hot.

Having said so much, let us now go over the ground again, and see how these actions are varied and regulated.

1. Our tastes for food are very various, enabling us to enjoy almost every kind, and to eat many kinds; and if any should not be at first agreeable, our tastes change, so that we begin to like them. Hence men can live under the most different conditions and with the greatest apparent diversity of food.

Our appetites also vary, but not in the same degree, for we need nearly the same quantity of food from day to day, and one man does not differ so very much from another.

The quantity of food required changes with the work which we do, and as our appetites also vary, we obtain the proper amount.

But although foods apparently differ in the greatest degree, they are very much alike in the kind of nourishment which they afford, so that they are easily classed together, and one member of a class can be taken instead of another. Thus bread, meat, and milk, have little similarity in appearance and taste, and yet they are made of similar things and perform the same kind of duties in the body. Again, fat, starch, and sugar seem very unlike each other, yet they are alike in their composition, and fat may be made from the others. In all these cases the quantity required may be different to produce the same result. Thus we have a great variety of foods by which our tastes are gratified, whilst they produce similar results in the body.

Foods require a certain time for digestion and distribution by the blood, and after that we again become hungry, and require more food. Hence we take a meal of various foods, and after several hours another, so that there are usually four hours between them, and three or four meals in the day. We do not take food during the night, and the food which had been taken and digested during the day is then perfectly disposed of, and ready to be cast out of the body.

As there is a long interval between supper and breakfast, most people enjoy their breakfast well, and the body then the most needs it. Therefore we should eat a good breakfast, and thus prepare to meet the wants of the day. About midday the working man has done a good deal of work, has consumed his breakfast, and wants another meal, and as he has still many hours' work to do he eats a good dinner, including meat when possible, which gives him the greatest amount of strength. After this, he has nearly done his work, and does not need much food, whilst the food already taken is still acting in him; and he eats a light meal at tea. His fourth meal depends upon the hour of the third, and the amount of food eaten and work done during the day, and may either be omitted or be a light one as his feelings indicate. As no work is done after supper, and many hours are spent in sleep, when digestion is very slowly performed, much food should not be eaten, or it will prevent sound sleep. Food should not be taken later than two hours before going to bed, and it should be of a light nature, as milk, and foods made of milk.

Such is the general rule of the working men in this country. The richer people dine at six to eight o'clock at night when it is really supper time, and eat only a little in the middle of the day when other people dine; but this would not be proper for working men who want a good meal of food at the time that they are doing work. It may suit those who work with their brains and not with their muscles, or those who do not work at all; but it would be better even for them to take a good lunch in the middle of the day, and a light and moderate dinner at supper time.

1. As to the quantity of food required every day. The best guide is the appetite when it is in a healthy state; but it is not well to eat until the appetite is fully satisfied lest we should feel oppressed and heavy with eating too much, but we should cease before that point is attained, and whilst still feeling fit to do our work. Infants and young children should, however, eat as much as they seem to want, and have more than four meals a day. Both infants and very old people also need food once or twice in the night.

2. As to digestion. This varies in rapidity with the different kinds of food; but it does not follow that because a food is rapidly digested it gives the most nourishment or is the best food. The usual time for the digestion of our ordinary food, as bread and meat, is from three to four hours, and then it leaves the stomach, and for some hours is circulating and acting in the blood. So it does not follow that a food which is slowly digested is a bad food, but if it requires more time than other foods it may be carried out of the stomach into the bowels before it is entirely digested, and be in part wasted. On the whole, therefore, foods which are digested very slowly are not so valuable as others, and hence pork and veal which require five, are not so good as mutton which is digested in three and a half hours. Perhaps also such as are quickly digested, as tripe, oysters, and fish, may not give us so much nutriment, but all that they can give us is extracted from them, and nothing is lost. Foods which are of very slow digestion satisfy the appetite for a longer time, so that the Indians in their long journeys being unable to obtain sufficient food, eat small balls of clay, which remain in the stomach and stop the appetite for many hours.

3. As to the circulation. As the circulation is intended to carry the blood through the body it will naturally

be the most rapid when the necessity is the greatest, and the least when it is not wanted. Thus after a meal it rapidly increases fifteen or twenty beats per minute for one and a half to two and a half hours, and then becomes gradually slower until the next meal, after which it rises and falls again. There is therefore an increase directly after every meal, and a decrease before the next meal. Generally the increase is the greatest after a good breakfast, and the least after supper. The pulsation is the lowest in the middle of the night, with sleep, at two to five o'clock in the winter, and one to three in the summer, and at that time many people who are very ill die.

These changes go on every day in all persons, but are the greatest in the young and least in the old. The greatest change, however, takes place with exertion, so that the number of beats may be doubled during great labour. Thus, when sitting at rest it may be sixty-four, walking at one mile per hour seventy-five, at two miles per hour eighty, at three miles per hour ninety, at four miles per hour one hundred and ten to one hundred and twenty, and running at six miles per hour one hundred and forty. This is in proportion to the waste of the muscles, and therefore to the necessity for food, and may be taken as a measure of the quantity of food which should be eaten under the different conditions referred to. But without exertion the difference between the lowest pulsations of the night and the highest after dinner may be thirty to fifty per minute.

4. As to the breathing. The breathing follows the same rule as the pulsation, although not necessarily in precisely the same degree, but it is the lowest in the night, has the same changes with meals, and is increased in nearly equal proportions by exertion.

5. As to producing heat. It is difficult to understand how

the digestion of a piece of bread and butter should yield heat, and yet we are familiar with some things which produce heat without flame or without being previously heated. Thus if oil of vitriol be added to water they become so hot that the hand cannot hold the glass containing them, and yet they were both cold before they were mixed. So by adding things of the same temperature together we can produce great cold. If sal ammoniac and common salt and water be added together they will produce cold enough to make ice from water. Hence, we ought to be able to admit that the mixture or combinations of things may produce heat. It is precisely so that the digestion and change of food within the body makes heat and warms it, and there is no chemical combination which has not the same result. This is called burning the food.

But different foods produce heat in very different degrees, and of them all fat generates the most, whilst meat produces more than bread or fruit. This explains the fact that fat is eaten in enormous quantities in very cold climates, meat in moderate quantities in all temperate regions, and vegetables and fruit in hot countries.

We are all conscious of being warm after a meal and cold when we are fasting, and the time when heat is produced to the greatest degree is during the digestion of food. Variation in heat corresponds with variation in pulsation and respiration; being, with rest, the least at night and the greatest after food, but with exertion increasing as the exertion increases. The coolness of the skin in sleep, the heat of the hands and face after a good meal, and the great sense of heat after violent exertion, are known to all.

But we have already stated that with all this the temperature of the inner parts of the body is nearly the same (say 99° to 101° Fah.) at all times. And how is this effected?

HEALTH.

The skin performs this function by causing increase of perspiration when the body is too hot, and lessening it when it is cool. A man at rest is cool and his skin has no perceptible moisture, but when he runs violently the perspiration trickles down his face, and his shirt becomes wet with it.

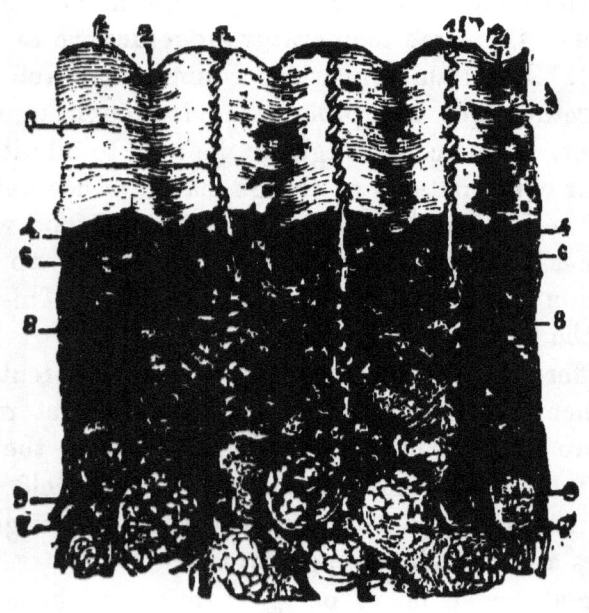

Fig. 41.

SECTION OF THE SKIN.

Fig. 41 shows a section of the skin with the minute structures which are necessary to its functions.

1, 2, and 3, The scarf skin, or epidermis.
8, The true skin.
4, Colouring matter of the skin.
6, Papillæ, by which we have the sense of touch.
7, Sweat glands, with ducts or tubes, 9, passing through the skin and scarf skin to the pores on the surface, 11, and throw out perspiration.

The explanation of the cooling of the body is easy to one who is acquainted with science. Fluids (like all other bodies) have heat in two forms, one of which is not perceptible, and is therefore called latent, and the other, which can be measured by the thermometer. A gas has 700 times more latent heat than a fluid, and when a fluid is converted into steam it absorbs all that additional heat, and makes the things about it colder. So when the water from the blood is poured out in perspiration and becomes steam it absorbs heat from the skin, and the skin becomes cooler. Thus the skin is the heat-regulator and offers a ready way of getting rid of unnecessary heat from the body by so simple an act as perspiring.

This goes on without our aid or will, but we afford some help by varying the amount of clothing and fuel as already mentioned.

Thus we see that food is the cause of nearly all the changes which occur in the body, and upon the proper supply and use of it health or disease chiefly depends.

CHAPTER X.

ATMOSPHERIC CONDITIONS.

We are surrounded by the atmosphere, and are influenced by all its variations night and day, so that it is necessary for us to take an account of it as it affects the question of health.

ELEMENTS OF THE ATMOSPHERE.

The air consists of two gases—oxygen and nitrogen—which are simply mixed together in the proportion of about twenty-one of the former to seventy-nine of the latter. There is also a small admixture of carbonic acid, and a quantity of vapour of water, which changes at every moment. These proportions vary somewhat in different places and at different times, as shown in the following table :—

TABLE

Showing the Proportion of Oxygen in 100 Parts of the Air on Mountains and the Ocean, in Cities, and many other Places.

1. *Mountains, Hills, and Seas.*

	Oxygen in 100 parts.
Gay-Lussac and Humboldt	20·9 to 21·2
,, in the air from mountains and fens .	21·49
De Saussure in the air from mountains . . .	20·98 to 21·15
Frankland in the air at Chamounix in Switzerland	20·80

	Oxygen in 100 parts.
Frankland in the air at the top of Mont Blanc	20·96
,, ,, near ,,	20·80
Miller in the air, 18,000 feet high, from a balloon	20·88
,, near the earth ,,	20·92
Dr. R. Angus Smith in the air on the tops of hills.	20·98
,, ,, ,, mountains in Scotland	20·98
,, at bottom of mountains in Scotland	20·94
,, in the air on the sea-shore in Scotland	20·99
Borgor, in the air, on Tara and other mountains	20·3 to 21·63
Brunner ,, Faulhorn	20·91
Regnault ,, on mountains higher than Mont Blanc	20·95 to 20·98
Regnault, in the air, of Ecuador	20·96
,, ,, on the Atlantic Ocean	20·92 to 20·96
Hermbstädt ,, on the Baltic Ocean	21·59
Vogel ,, ,,	21·59

2. *Cities.*

Dr. R. Angus Smith, in the air of London:—	
N., N.E., and N.W. districts average	20·85
S. and S.W. ,,	20·88
E. and E.C. ,,	20·86
W.C. and W. ,,	20·92
N.W., S., S.W., and W., &c.	20·95
Many open places in summer	20·95
Worst parts of Perth	20·93
Many parts of Scotland	20·96
Dalton, in the air of Manchester	20·7 to 21·15
Regnault ,, Paris	average 20·95
,, ,, ,,	20·91 to 20·99
,, ,, Lyons and neighbourhood	20·91 to 20·96
,, ,, Berlin	20·90 to 20·99
,, ,, Madrid	20·91 to 20·98
,, ,, Geneva	20·90 to 20·99
,, ,, Toulon	20·91 to 20·98
Bunsen ,, Heidelberg (average)	20·84 to 20·92

Of the two gases, nitrogen is useful only to dilute and mix with the oxygen, for it does not act as food or upon food. We may therefore omit any further reference to it.

Oxygen is that element without which food could not be

made useful to the body, and upon which strength, heat, and even life, depend. It is taken into the lungs by breathing, and there absorbed into the blood vessels, by which it is carried to all parts of the system. Whilst performing this journey it is always acting, and unites with hydrogen to form water, and with carbon to form carbonic acid, both of which are thrown out of the body by expiration; besides making many other compounds which pass out by the skin and kidneys. When a spark is placed in oxygen it breaks out into a flame, whilst a piece of heated wire burns and phosphorus is ignited in it, and an additional proportion of it in the air increases the effects of respiration. Hence it maintains heat, light, and life, but when added to hydrogen it forms water, and to carbon, carbonic acid, and these useful properties are lost, so that in both of them an animal dies, and a flame goes out. It is in forming this union that oxygen gives out heat, and, most of all, in its combination with hydrogen. It ceases to have any further power so long as that union continues, but when it is again free it can sustain heat, light, and life, as before. Thus it is essential to health that it exist in a sufficient proportion in the atmosphere, that it be breathed, that it undergo these changes, that it be thrown out of the body, and that it be again set free.

As to the first, it will be in the proper quantity if no other gas has been added to atmospheric air, but if otherwise, it will be so much less as the other is present. This other gas is almost always the carbonic acid produced by respiration, or the burning of gas, candles, coal, or any other substance, and in proportion as it is present the air becomes unfit for respiration, and tends to cause disease. As to the second it varies with the rapidity and depth of respiration, and we have seen how greatly that changes with food and exertion. The third is more constant, but whilst it increases or diminishes health as it occurs, it is lessened by a state of ill-health, and increased by perfect health.

The fourth takes place with the second, for the expiration is the same in amount as the inspiration, and the quantities of each are practically equal. But then arises the question of the removal of this foul air so that it may not be again breathed. This may be effected in two ways: first, by the person walking away from it, as when he takes exercise in the open air; and secondly, by the air being carried away by bringing in fresh air, or, as it is called, ventilation. Whenever a person breathes in a room which is closed he must in time breathe some of the same air over again; but if there be openings, so as to cause a current of air, some of that which he has breathed will be carried away, and fresh air will be brought in. This is the same whether the openings be doors, windows, chimney flues, or special ventilators, and its sufficiency will depend upon the quantity of foul air expired and the rapidity of its removal. The quantity of foul air will depend chiefly upon the number of persons breathing air, or the amount of gas burning in the room. The quantity of air admitted will depend upon the number and size of the openings, and the rapidity of the current, and it will therefore be increased or diminished by the direction and force of the wind.

There are also two other forces to be mentioned. Heat, by expanding the air, makes it lighter, and causes it to rise, and thus displaces and removes any given quantity, and is a very important agent in ventilation. The other is the property, which all gases have, of mixing with each other, so that a whiff of tobacco-smoke brought into a room will, in a short time, spread to every part. This is called universal diffusion, and is ever, yet slowly, acting, and tends to remove a part of a particular gas from one place to another.

Upon the proper consideration of these questions depends nearly the whole science of ventilation, and the art is the more difficult inasmuch as rooms, people, winds, and heat vary in every house and at every moment. It is quite clear that it must differ with the season, and also that an amount of ventilation which would be sufficient for a very few per-

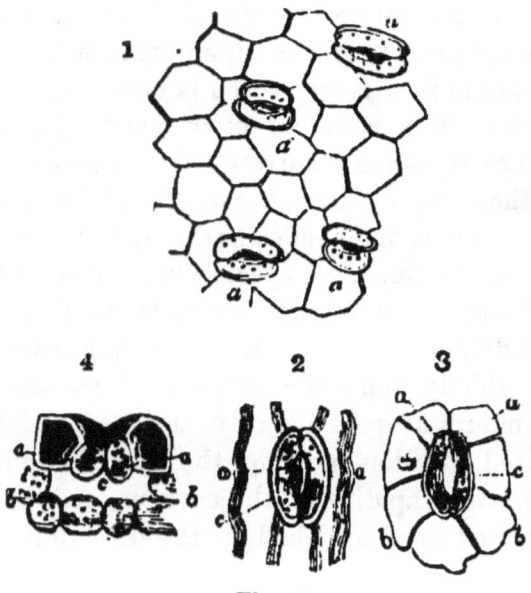

Stomata, or Mouths of Plants.

Fig. 42.

sons in a room, would be quite inadequate if the number were greatly increased.

As to the fifth, the mode by which the oxygen is again freed from the carbonic acid is by the respiration of vegetables, which live upon the carbon, and under the influence of the sunlight separate the oxygen, and set it free into the atmosphere, as shown by the beautiful Stomata of Plants in Figure 42. These little mouths, by which plants breathe air and drink in moisture, are found chiefly on the underside of the leaves. They are seen in their natural state at 1, 2, and 3, whilst in 4 one has been cut through to show the chamber into which it opens on the inside of the leaf. Hence, wherever much carbonic acid is made, there should be vegetables to unmake it. But it is made chiefly in great towns, where numbers of people live, and where there can be no vegetation near. Here, then, we have another necessity for the winds, which move the air, and carry town air to the country and the sea, and bring country air to the towns. When there is very little or no movement of the air, the atmosphere in great towns becomes foul and oppressive, and causes disease. This is seen in July and August, when, with much heat and little wind, everybody in London becomes weak and oppressed, and, under certain conditions, fever, diarrhœa, and cholera prevail. But with strong winds and storms all the foul air is dispersed, the atmosphere becomes fresh, and we are invigorated, cheerful, and well.

Heat has great influence over the atmosphere, because as the air is expanded, there is less oxygen in the same volume, and therefore less oxygen is inspired by us, whilst, as it contracts by cold, more oxygen is inspired. The former lessens vital changes, and the latter increases them; and it is well known that we are stronger and feel more able to work with mind and body in cool than in hot weather. In this respect, however, we have a great advantage in our temperate climate, for it is never too hot nor too cold to prevent work; whilst in very hot and very cold climates, there is less work performed. Moreover, violent and sudden changes in either direction soon bring on storms, which restore the normal state. An extremely hot day in spring, with the wind from the south, will soon take the wind to the south-west or some other cooler quarter, and bring rain. This is by far the most important cause of winds, and, disagreeable as it may be, it also brings us relief.

PRESSURE.

The weight of the atmosphere is about fifteen pounds on every square inch, or thirty thousand pounds on the whole of our body, and therefore enough to crush us to the ground if the atmosphere did not press upon us equally on all sides, and thereby enable us to keep upright as easily as to lie down. But variations in the weight have a marked influence upon our feeling of health, and upon the action of our bodies, both within and without. The changes are shown by the barometer, so that it stands at about 30 inches (or sustains a column of mercury 30 inches high), when the weight of the column of air is about 15 lbs. on the square inch, rising when the air is heavier, and falling when it is lighter. The barometer is commonly high with dry and frosty, and low in wet, weather; and has such an influence upon us, that we are comparatively strong and cheerful with a high, and weak and dispirited with a low, state of the instrument.

The following are the principal effects of the varying pressure upon the body:—

With a high barometer or great pressure,—

1. The circulation is supported and quickened.
2. The air is condensed, so that we breathe more oxygen in a given volume, and have more vital action.
3. The outflow of water by the kidneys is increased, whilst that of the skin is lessened.
4. Our appetite for food is increased.
5. Our capability for work is increased.
6. Our spirits are commonly higher.

With a low barometer, the reverse of these effects may be expected, and our spirits, circulation, appetite, and vital changes languish; whilst we have less power to make exertion, and there is a greater tendency to perspire and to take cold.

Whenever the barometer falls very low, we are conscious of something unusual in the state of the atmosphere, which leads those to look at that instrument whose duty it is to watch changes in the weather, as sailors at sea; and although a storm may be expected, these sensations occur some time before there is any appearance of such a change. So also on a bright frosty morning, when the wind is still, and the barometer high, we are strong and cheerful, and ready for any exertion; and although some of this feeling is due to the cold, it is partly due also to the increased pressure of the atmosphere. A high barometer is a more healthful and happy sign than a low one.

MOISTURE.

The atmosphere, in every part and at all times, contains a quantity of watery vapour, which, when it is deposited, becomes dew. The quantity is increased by raising the temperature, and decreased by lowering it; for there is a limit to the quantity of vapour which air can contain. When the air is full, it is said to be saturated, and any quantity beyond that is deposited as dew. But let the air be then heated, and it is no longer saturated, and will contain more; and even with more, may be really drier than before, for it may be able to carry a yet greater quantity of vapour. Let such be now made cooler, and although it may still have the same quantity of vapour, it will be less dry, for it is nearer to saturation and to the point when it will deposit it. These are very familiar facts to us. Let a glass of lukewarm water be brought into a warm room, and no change will appear upon it, but let a glass of cold or iced water be brought, and it soon becomes covered with moisture from the air immediately about it. Go into a field on a clear night, and you may find dew on a stone but not on a piece of wood; and the reason is that the stone radiates heat quicker than the wood, and by that means cools the air about it, and causes it to be saturated and to deposit moisture.

Hence air is dry or moist, not according to the weight of vapour which it has in a given volume, but according to its temperature, and therefore to the capacity which it has to receive more vapour. A wind blowing over a hot desert or sandy plain becomes drier, not because the sand has taken moisture from it, but because it has become hotter and could absorb a greater quantity than it had before. Let such a wind then blow over the sea and it takes up a quantity of vapour, and becomes lower in temperature and is again moist. Thus our easterly winds are dry, whilst our south-westerly are wet; the former being far from saturated, whilst the latter may be nearly saturated, and require only a small fall of temperature to cause the vapour to fall as rain.

The importance of this to health is extreme. Thus we lose a great part of the water which we have drank by the expired air, since the air is of higher temperature than the atmosphere, and is also saturated. The drier, therefore, the air which we breathe, the greater will be the quantity of vapour which it can carry from the body. Now if we breathed air as hot as our bodies and yet saturated, no water could leave by expiration, and we should be oppressed and faint. On the other hand, if we breathed air at the same high temperature, which was extremely dry, it would carry off a great quantity of vapour, and we should be better or worse, as we could lose the vapour with advantage. These changes are seen in the Turkish and the steam-bath. In the former, the hot air is very dry and carries off much vapour from the lungs, whilst in the latter the air is fully charged and cannot absorb any more.

It has also the same effect over the skin, and either prevents or greatly increases the perspiration. To be surrounded by hot and saturated air in hot weather prevents the cooling of the body by the lungs, and a sense of faintness occurs, with or without fever, as is seen in many hot countries and occasionally in our own in close and damp valleys.

Hence health, and even life, depend upon this quality of dryness or moisture of the atmosphere which we breathe or which surrounds us. This shows the reason for change of climate and season.

As to season. In winter the air is cool and near to saturation, but as we warm the air by respiration it becomes dry and we lose vapour. Hence respiration and the cooling of the body are then free; and as the winds are strong the air is freely circulated and we get good air and are invigorated. At that period there is the greatest vital action in the body and the highest degree of health and fitness for the duties of life. In summer the heat is greater and the quantity of vapour which can be carried off by respiration is less; and should the air be both hot and moist we cannot cool the body. The air is generally still and sometimes stagnant, and therefore not fresh and pure. At that season, say in August, the vital actions are the least, and we have less muscular vigour and less disposition and ability to work. Then we are liable to the most mortal diseases, and our only relief is in the violent storms which excess of heat induces, after which we say that the air is cool and fresh.

The spring is the most healthful of all the seasons, because it follows a cool season, and we have none of the extremes of the others, and yet we have the highest state of the vital actions and strong winds. We have no difficulty in cooling the body, whilst the appetite enables us to eat plenty of food and thus to produce much heat and to perform all our physical duties perfectly.

The autumn is much less healthful because it follows the depressing influences of summer, and has the air often laden with moisture. The temperature and winds are very uncertain, and when the former is high and the latter quiet, disease of the nature of fever and exhaustion is sure to prevail. Hence it has been taught in all ages that autumn is the period of the year when there is the greatest danger to health, and when the greatest care is required to prevent colds and to maintain the full vigour of the body.

ELECTRICITY.

An electrical or "thundery" state of the atmosphere has always a depressing influence, and in many persons causes profuse perspiration, fainting, and loss of appetite and spirits. Every one feels that there is a difference in the air before and after a thunder-storm, and it is due partly to the discharge of the electricity by lightning, and partly to the violent rain and wind which often accompany it. When the air is very warm, close, and stifling, and there is much distant lightning, we do not feel relief until the discharges come near and bring a storm.

The great power of electricity is well known, for it splits the trunks of trees, breaks down high church spires, and kills men and animals. It should also be known to every one that it strikes the highest object, provided it be a tree, or a building having iron in its construction, and therefore no one should take shelter under a tree when the lightning is very near. You will know how distant it is by observing the interval of time between the flash and the thunder, for whilst the flash is seen instantly, sound travels in air at about a mile in $4\frac{3}{4}$ seconds, and you hear the thunder after you have seen the flash, although both occurred together. All high buildings should have lightning conductors of thin rods of iron projecting above them, to draw the electricity from the clouds and carry it to the earth without producing a flash of lightning.

LIGHT.

The use of light is extremely great, and the pleasure which it gives is beyond expression. What do the Esquimaux think of it when for many months in the year they are in total darkness; and how gladly do they get to the top of the highest hills to see the first return of the sun, which shall give them light by both day and night for some of the other months!

How does the plant growing in a cellar seem to long for light when it turns and stretches itself towards the opening in the shutter through which a gleam of light enters! Such a plant would be green and strong if it grew in the light, but in darkness it is whitish-yellow, thin, and weak.

So with the poor children who are brought up in the close, dark courts and underground cellars in some of our large towns. They grow up pale, thin, weak, and spiritless, or die at a very early age. Those who live in the open air and run in green fields should be very thankful for their advantages, and consider how useful, agreeable, and beautiful a thing is light.

Light is necessary for the proper growth of both animals and plants, and for the restoration to the atmosphere of the oxygen which we have elsewhere said is locked up in the carbonic acid from respiration, until it is set free by plants. In those northern countries where is no light for many months at a time, there are no plants such as we see here, and the animals and inhabitants are extremely few, and do not much increase in numbers.

Light may exert greater action on the body than we are aware of, but its effect upon our spirits is well known; and how should we be acquainted with the beauties of nature if we had it not? We should be dull and mopish, ignorant and stupid, even if we could live, in continual darkness. But the amount of it varies with the season, so that there is much more light in summer than winter, because the sun then rises higher in the heavens, and there is commonly less cloud. So it varies with climate, and in some places it is so great that they are glad to live in darkened rooms to escape from it when it is the brightest, or to wear dark-coloured spectacles. Have we not, even in England, sometimes been thankful for a cloud to hide the sun on a burning summer day, and to protect us not only from the great heat, but from the light? Have you ever considered how beautiful and useful are the clouds, with their varying shapes, densities, and colours, and what our atmosphere would be in summer with great light and heat and a bare blue sky above us?

With too much light the skin becomes bleached, and we lose the ruddy glow of health, whilst disease of the eyes is often caused in those unhealthy children who are liable to scrofulous diseases.

On considering these statements about the atmosphere we must see the great advantage of the changes which take place in our sea-girt island and climate, and, instead of complaining, should be thankful that we live under conditions which are more favourable to health than any other people in the world. Those nations who have extremely cold winters for seven or eight months in the year, as in Canada, or who have extremely hot and dry weather for many months without change, as in India, or who have a season of continued rain for two or three months, would be delighted with our changes, by which sunshine and showers, heat and cold, dry and wet, are wonderfully mingled together, and give us so great a variety of pleasure and pain. Only let us enjoy the good, and try to avoid the evil, and be thankful.

CHAPTER XI.

THE MIND, AND MENTAL WORK.

THERE are some who thoughtlessly say that the condition of the mind has nothing to do with the health of the body; but although the connection is not so distinct as that between food and health, it is nevertheless real and powerful. It is true that many have apparently robust health who take no pains to cultivate and direct their minds; but, on the other hand, it is equally true that those who perform much mental work frequently fall into serious bodily disease. It may be allowed that defective cultivation of the mind may still leave the body in full power to work, and thus reduce man to the level of the lower animals; but better cultivation of the mind might yet save the body from many diseases into which it falls, and enable it to do better and more useful work. As the body is directed, so it may be protected, by the mind, and either kept from danger or be more quickly restored to a state of sanity.

How many colds are taken without consideration, and how many diseases are brought on by idleness and intemperance, which would have been avoided if the man had had the resource of a cultivated mind! How many improper or dangerous foods are eaten for the want of knowledge, and how many accidents (so called) happen which with more intelligence and observation might have been avoided! A well-cultivated and regulated mind is not only no hindrance to the full development of the powers of the body but may greatly aid them.

Take, however, on the other hand, the case of a youth who is exceedingly studious, and falls into disease. Is the result due to the cultivation of the mind, or to the neglect of the most reasonable precautions as to bodily health? He sits up late at night, bends over his books, takes too little exercise, eats too little food, has languor and indigestion, looks pale and thin, and is weak and ready to fall into consumption. All this may be true, but is not necessary; and, on the contrary, however he may have cultivated his mind in some directions, it shows clearly that he has failed in that which people call common sense, and has thereby injured both body and mind.

Hence the cultivation of the mind should be carried on with judgment, and in due submission to the requirements of the body. If study be the duty of the youth, let him pursue it diligently, but with such intervals of rest and bodily exertion as may maintain good appetite and health.

The proportion of hours of study and bodily exercise may vary with the degree of mental work, the healthfulness of the room and surrounding air, the natural strength of the body and the degree of health; but as a general rule it may be doubted whether any young person can sit at close study for more than two hours at a time without requiring bodily exertion to sustain vital action, and rest to recruit the mind. Two hours' mental work and a quarter to half an hour's bodily exercise, will be quite compatible with the greatest progress in study.

Moreover, it may be doubted whether such a student can work with advantage for more than eight hours a day, in addition to the intervals of rest; for the issue will not turn upon the number of hours devoted to work, but upon the intensity of the attention given, and the complete appreciation of the subject. It is much more easy to study in a dreamy fashion than in earnest; and to read a little and then think of other things, than to fix the mind earnestly upon one thing for a period of two hours.

Again; whilst many may be unable to rise at 4 or 5 A.M. to study, or if they do rise, are scarcely awake, it is no doubt much more useful to employ the early rather than the later hours of the day for that purpose. Four or five hours spent in mental work before mid-day will yield far better results than those which may be spent afterwards, and have the further advantage of leaving time for bodily and mental recreation, after a proper day's work shall have been done.

There are many who affirm that they work the most satisfactorily after midnight, but such are exceptions to a rule, and probably work less well at an earlier part of the day by reason of ill-arranged meals or other habits. Such a condition is not desirable.

But what shall we say to those who must follow another occupation during the day, and cultivate their minds when that has ended? They deserve greater credit than those whose duty it is to cultivate their minds all the day, and should not be discouraged. A large majority of occupations are such as need not exhaust the mind or greatly fatigue the body in their pursuit, so that there may be no real difficulty in devoting two or three hours in the evening to mental cultivation; and to many such a change brings real relaxation. Let them occupy an hour before the morning labour, when it is possible, and thus shorten the work at night by an hour, and they will find study less onerous, and any supposed evil effect upon the body a myth. There is no reason to believe that study during one such morning hour and two hours at night will injure, provided the health be fairly good and the surroundings healthful. Let such young men take courage, and remember that some of the most distinguished men have laboriously obtained their fame under difficulties as great as theirs.

Hence the cardinal rules of health are:—

1. Work in the early, rather than in the later, part of the day, and do not rob yourself of sleep before midnight.

2. Alternate your mental work with bodily relaxation, and make as much use of the latter as the time will allow. Gymnastics, which expand the chest, singing, shouting, running, and jumping, are proper kinds of relaxation.

3. Limit your mental toil to that number of hours which will enable you to work well with the mind, and to obtain proper recreation for the body, as well as facilities of observation for the mind.

One great advantage of the cultivation of the mind in its relation to health, in addition to the increased intelligence which is thus acquired, is a sense of satisfaction and ease of conscience, by which the pleasures of life are enhanced and enjoyed. Whatever enables a man to have a conscience void of offence towards God and towards man, should lead to health, and although this is not the highest, it is one of the higher grounds on which such a desirable result is based. We too much neglect the cultivation of that part of our nature which is immortal, and attend to that which presses its claims more urgently, and yet is perishable. A happy and intelligent man, other things being equal, should be a more healthy man than he who lives a careless animal life only.

In connection with this subject is that quality or condition which we call spirits; and can we doubt that good spirits do wait upon good appetite, digestion and health, whilst low spirits represent languor and disease? These are due partly to nature, for some have as naturally a flow of good spirits as others are melancholy, mopish, and low-spirited, and it becomes each to endeavour to reach the happy medium; partly to the weather, for a fine, bright, sunny day cheers, whilst a gloomy, dark, and cold day dispirits every one; but, above all, to the due regulation of the mind, and a conscientious discharge of the duties of life. An even flow of spirits is as conducive to our own health as to the happiness of those around us, and should be diligently cultivated and jealously guarded.

CHAPTER XII.

THE SPECIAL SENSES.

THE EYE.

THE eye differs much in structure as it is seen in a fly and in the higher animals, but that of man and the higher animals is the same, and is the most perfect of any known to us. It consists of a dark chamber enclosed by very strong tissues to protect it from accidental injury, and lined by the retina or expanded nerve which receives the impression of the rays of light, and through the optic nerve conveys them to the mind.

The light is admitted into this chamber from the front of the eye and in such quantities as the pupil will allow.

First, it passes through the outer structure called the cornea (Fig. 44), (covered by the mucous membrane or conjunctiva), which consists of several layers, all of which are transparent when healthy, but in a state of disease may become opaque as is seen in the white specks on many eyes. It then enters into a chamber in which hangs the curtain called the iris, of a different colour in the eyes of different persons, and passes through it by the opening called the pupil (Fig. 43). This important part is made larger or smaller by the degree of contraction of the iris, and then admits many rays or excludes all but those which pass through the centre of it. It is larger when the light is feeble as at night, and smaller when the light is very strong, and admits a proportionate amount of light into the eye. It corresponds also with the state of the general health; for one who is weak has a pupil which is larger than when he is well; and also with the condition of the brain, for in inflammation of the brain and in certain states of madness it becomes contracted almost to a pin's point.

This curtain (Fig. 43) hangs in a fluid called the aqueous or watery humour, which varies in amount in different persons, as will be stated presently, and by which the cornea is made to project forward to a greater or less extent (Fig. 44.)

The next important structure is the crystalline lens (Fig. 44), which, like the cornea consists of layers, and is transparent in health; but in disease—called cataract—or by old age it becomes opaque. It is doubly convex—that is somewhat rounded in form, but is more expanded towards the back than the front of the eye, so that it may distribute the rays of light over the whole surface of the retina, but it is so constructed that it makes the rays converge towards a certain point. When it is opaque it prevents the light passing through it, or so hinders it that objects are seen very indistinctly, and should it be opaque in the direct line of the pupil but not on the side, the person may see, with the direction of the image changed.

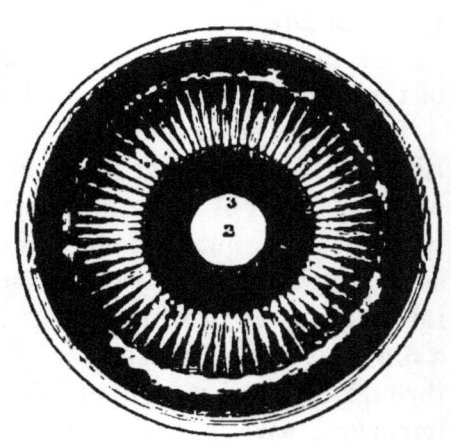

Fig. 43.
THE IRIS.

The iris, 3, is seen from the inner side of the eye, having the ciliæ, 4, and the pupil, 2.

The importance of this structure is therefore extremely

great, whether in assisting or preventing sight. When it is opaque it must be removed by an operation, after which doubly convex spectacles are used, and the person can again see. The lens is thus practically transferred from the inside to the outside of the eye.

The lens may be readily examined by boiling the eye of a sheep or other animal in water, for it falls out like a white marble when the eye is cut open. It can also be seen in its transparent state when a fresh eye is carefully opened without allowing the contents to escape. It can be crushed between the thumb and finger and then the central part is found to be more solid than the surface.

Immediately behind the lens, and occupying all the remaining part of the chamber, is the vitreous or glassy humour, which is of a greenish hue and something like jelly, but allows the rays of light to pass freely through it. If by any accident much of this fluid is lost the sight is seriously injured; but the fluid in the anterior chamber immediately behind the cornea may be let out without injury, as in the operation for cataract, for it will be again secreted and the eye become as useful as before.

There are many other structures in the eye which are known to anatomists and liable to disease, but it is not necessary for our purpose to describe them, and it is only requisite to add that the image of an object which is thrown upon the retina is inverted or upside down, and not erect as the object exists in nature. This may be shown by taking an ox's eye and carefully cutting out a portion at the back, when the image of an object which has passed through the lens is seen upside down;—or yet more easily, by clearing the back of the eye of a white rabbit and placing a lighted object in front, when the inverted image will be seen.

The structures which have thus been described are delineated in Fig. 44.

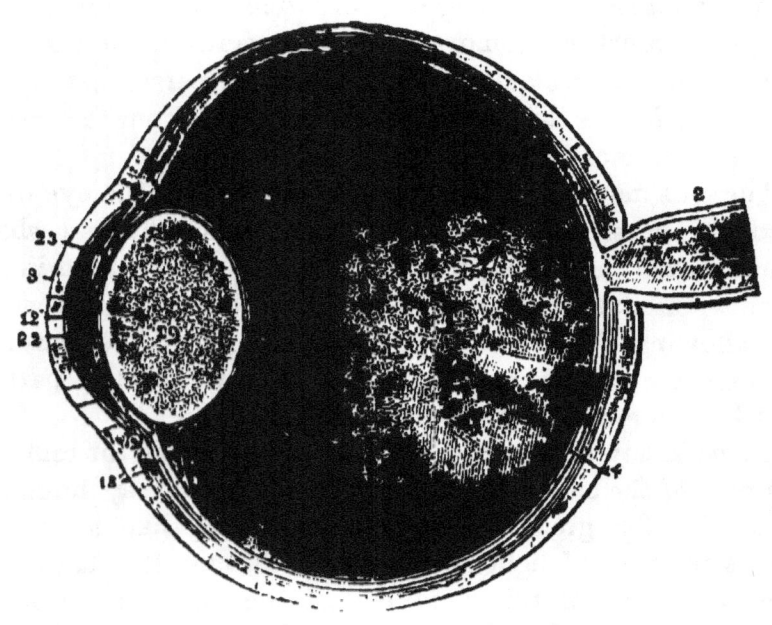

Fig. 44.
SECTION OF THE EYE.

1, The optic nerve enclosed in its sheath, 2.
19, The lens through which the light passes to enter the vitreous humour, 18, and to make its impressions upon the retina, 14.
23, The iris with the pupil, 12.
3, The cornea, or transparent structure forming the front of the eye.
22, The anterior chamber filled with water.

This organ is liable to two very common defects, viz., long sight and short sight, to which it may be desirable to briefly refer, as well as to numerous diseases which cannot be described here.

Short and long sight mean that an object is not seen in the most perfect degree at the distance from the eye at which it is well seen by mankind generally, viz., at about sixteen inches. A short-sighted person holds his book nearer, it may be, quite near to the eye, whilst the long-sighted holds it at a distance of two feet or upwards. This is due to the quantity of water in the anterior chamber of the eye, by which, in the case of short sight, the front of the eye, or the cornea, is made too round or projecting, and in the long sight too flat. Both are remedied by proper spectacles, so that with each defect objects may be seen at the usual distance.

The cause of this is sometimes a natural one, for the eye of the young is fuller, and after middle life flatter, so that the former tends to short, and the latter to long sight ; but both, and the former more particularly, is not unfrequently due to the habit of holding the object unnecessarily close to the eye, or of lowering the head very near to the object. Drawing and fine needle-work very commonly lead to it, as also the habit of doing such work with an insufficient amount of light, by which the object and the eye are made to approach each other. This is sometimes the result of carelessness, but much more frequently of ignorance ; and it becomes all those who have charge of youth to watch these habits with attention, and correct them at once.

Their importance is extremely great, for a short-sighted person is unable to see and appreciate the beauties of nature, frequently falls into error from imperfect observation, and not unfrequently gives offence to those who are not recognised when within the ordinary limits of recognition. It is perhaps more common among girls than boys, and leads to defective education. So soon as it is discovered (and it often remains undiscovered for years) spectacles should be obtained, and proper efforts made to extend the focus more and more by withdrawing the head from the object. Those having this defect who attain to middle life commonly lose it (if they do not wear spectacles which are needlessly strong) as age advances.

Those who have long sight are unable to see minute objects when very near, and therefore not only do not see the beauties visible to others, but cannot determine whether an object looks the same to others as to themselves. The former may be remedied by the use of spectacles, but the latter evil is never entirely removed.

It should therefore be the aim of all persons to ascertain whether their sight is natural, and if it be not, to have it corrected by judicious practice and the use of spectacles; always, however, taking care that the latter shall be somewhat weaker than the occasion requires, so that the short-sighted may ere long see properly without spectacles; and the long-sighted should increase the power of their spectacles very slowly with the increasing defects of age.

This is not a proper occasion on which to refer to diseases of the eye generally, but two are so common and important, that they demand some notice.

SQUINTING.

Squinting not only deforms and distorts the features of a child but interferes with the direction of vision, and therefore with the use of the eye. The eye affected is rarely so perfect an instrument of sight as the other, and the longer the obliquity remains the more the evil progresses. As it is more difficult to bring objects within proper grasp, imperfect and erroneous impressions are produced.

The cause, when squinting is simple, and not dependent upon prior disease of the eye, is the undue contraction of one or more of the muscles of the eyeball, by which the centre of the eye is drawn out of the proper line of vision. When it arises from this a small operation will immediately remove it, and it cannot be removed by any other means.

OPHTHALMIA IN SCHOOLS.

Inflammatory diseases of the eye are very common among the children of the poor. This is partly due to disease in infancy, partly to a diseased constitution, and partly to the habit of rubbing the eyes with dirty hands when there is an itching sensation. Parents may not be able to remedy the first two without the aid of the surgeon, but the third may be prevented by constant watchfulness and cleanliness, and by attention to the directions which will now be given for children living in schools.

The fact that Ophthalmia prevails in our large schools cannot be denied, and the injury which it inflicts upon the children in their prospects in life can scarcely be overstated; but the causes are more numerous and deeper seated than is generally supposed, and the disease itself when established is very intractable. Many of the causes, however, are preventible, and the authorities are not always without blame in reference to them.

The first and most important cause is not within the control of the authorities, viz., the constitutional state of the children on admission. Disease of a scrofulous character is very common amongst the poor of our agricultural districts, and that of the eyes not less frequent than of the joints, but it is not simply a local disease, since it is due primarily to a defect in the general health. Such children, moreover, have been underfed and exposed to many unsanitary conditions, whilst at the same time the treatment of their disease has been neglected.

These children when admitted into the schools suffer, or have suffered, from this diseased state of the system if not of the eyes, and however treated will be liable to a recurrence throughout youth—as many years probably as they will remain in the school. The next series of causes are, however, preventible, and demaud much more attention than they have received. Take the following:—

The school-room is almost always ill-ventilated, often over-crowded, with the temperature higher than that of other rooms, whilst the air is close, stagnant, and irritating from the exhalations of the bodies of the children. This renders every part of the body, and particularly the eyes, which are uncovered, unduly sensitive, whilst the children have their tone of health lowered still further, and are thereby more likely to fall into disease. When the school tasks are over the children rush into and about the play-ground, which is probably exposed to every point of the compass, and to a cold north-easterly as readily as to a warm southerly wind, by which the sensitive eye becomes congested or inflamed. In numerous instances the surface of the playground is covered with gravel or sand, and the feet and wind together throw volumes of gritty dust into the air which lodge in the eyes and further inflame them.

Play over, the children go into the lavatory, which is very cold and damp, and there wash in cold water, with the aid of common acrid soap, which gets under the lids and further irritates the eyes. When the child with smarting eyes wishes to dry the soap and water away, he uses a towel which is already wet and unable to absorb water, and therefore rubs away at his face and eyes in the vain hope of ridding himself of the nuisance. Probably the towel has been used by others having the disease, and is soiled with the diseased secretions, and may actually communicate the disease to a healthy child.

Further, the dining-room is generally overcrowded and hot, and full of the fumes of dinner, which may produce some degree of irritation in the eyes, and after staying there for twenty minutes the children rush into the playground as they did from the schoolroom.

The bedrooms in all the modern pauper schools are large, airy, and very cold, both by reason of the amount of space which is now demanded for each child and the absence of any method of warming them. Nothing is more common than to hear the officials in charge complain of this, as it respects the young children in the cold weather. Lofty, long, and wide rooms, with a separate bed for each child, and no distribution of heat, can have no other effect in the winter; and when the children leave their beds in the morning and dress and go into the cold lavatory, they are the very impersonation of cold.

Moreover, whilst the dietary, taken as a whole, may be sufficient, it is ill distributed, since there are but three meals a-day allowed, and if the meat which is given at one meal were distributed over several, it would nourish the children better. A child does not need four ounces or five ounces of cooked meat at a meal, but it requires four meals a day, which instead of being cold or lukewarm should be hot. Gruel and pea-soup are also as much too freely, as milk is stintingly, supplied.

What then is necessary in reference to preventible causes?

1. To prevent an undue elevation of temperature in some of the rooms, and thereby the sudden changes from heat to cold;

2. To warm in a moderate degree the lavatories and bedrooms;

3. To prevent gritty dust in the playgrounds, and to provide play sheds not exposed to the north and east winds;

4. To supply good white curd soap and chilled water, and a larger quantity of towels, taking care to dry the wet towels if not sufficiently dirty to be removed.

5. To regulate the dietary more in accordance with home feeding.

In addition there should be a system of special supervision of those children who are of a scrofulous habit and peculiarly liable to ophthalmia.

In reference to treatment, it is clear that the first duty is to separate the diseased from the healthy, and to supply to each individual that warmth and food, soap, water, and towels which his case requires, and to add the treatment of the general health and of the eyes, which every medical man knows how to apply to such cases. Needless spreading of the disease will be prevented by such means, although the constitution and local conditions may not be very amenable to treatment, and the case may linger long in hospital.

It is also clear that the medical officer should pass before all the children in the school in single file at least once a week, and carefully notice the state of the eyes and the general health; whilst if there were medical inspectors of the central authority they would be able to confer with the local medical officer, to the advantage of the school.

We again say that more injury is caused by bad soap and wet towels than is generally believed. All these evils may not exist in every school, or in an equal degree, but they do exist and are nearly universal.

THE EAR.

The ear, like the eye, does not differ in man and the higher animals, but is the most perfect in them, and infinitely more so than the same organ in fishes and the lower animals.

It consists of three parts essential for collecting and transmitting sound, and for producing the sense of hearing, which are represented in the four following beautiful figures.

THE EAR.

The outer ear, or auricle, is so formed that it collects the vibrations of the air and directs them to the middle ear. This effect is readily understood by placing the half closed hand at the back of the ear, by which the vibrations are collected in a further degree, and hearing is increased. On the other hand, when the ear is flattened to the head or the hollow of it is filled up, the sense of hearing is lessened; and as the size and form of the ear vary in different persons, the sense of hearing must vary also.

The tube or auditory canal which leads from the outer to the middle ear begins at the outside and ends on the inside with the tightly stretched membrane called the drum. It becomes narrower as it goes inwards, and is directed inward and forward, but is not perfectly direct in its course or even in its form. It is surrounded by bone which receives some of the vibrations of the air and assists the sense of hearing; and when the tube is filled, as by the finger, sounds are heard in the head which are conveyed by the bony structures, and were not heard before.

There are hairs at the entrance of the tube to arrest the admission of dust and other substances, and wax is secreted in the tube which may so increase as to fill it, and produce the same sounds as when the finger is placed in the ear. The quantity of hairs does not give rise to any inconvenience, but that of wax is important and leads to the habit of picking the ear, to which reference will again be made. When it is insufficient it is usually the result of disease, and when too abundant should be removed by injecting warm water into the tube. The tube is lined by a membrane which may be inflamed and thickened to the injury of the sense of hearing.

The drum is somewhat oval in form, attached to bone at its edges, and lying obliquely across the tube. It is moved by the vibrations of the air somewhat as in an ordinary drum by the strokes of a stick, and conveys them to the inner ear, by a very small bone which is attached to its centre. Its use is therefore to intensify and convey the

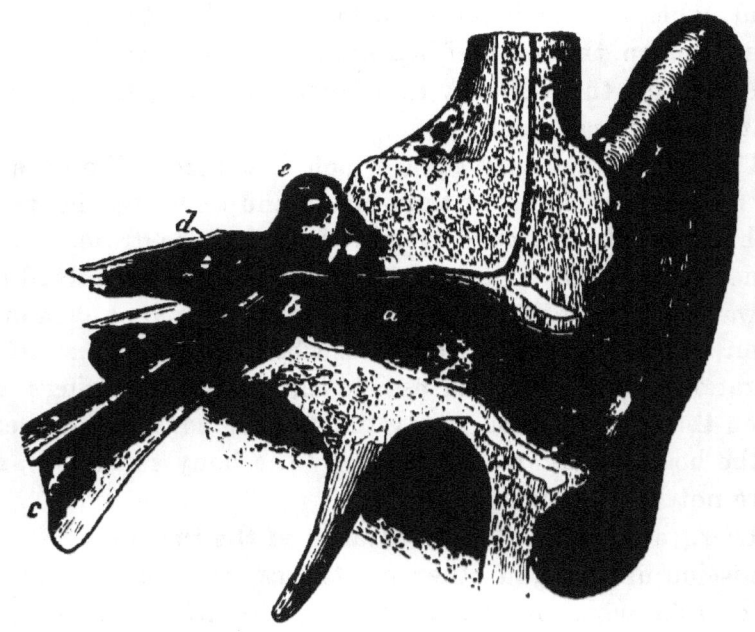

Fig. 45.

SECTION OF THE HUMAN EAR.

a, The external tube ending at the drum, and surrounded by bone.
b, The inner end of the eustachian tube, ending at the drum.
c, The commencement of the eustachian tube in the throat.
e and *d*, The inner ear or the semi-circular canals and cochlea.

vibrations of the air to that part by which they will be felt and hearing produced, and it is said to divide the outer from the middle ear.

The above figure shows the parts already described, and also a tube which begins on the inner side of the drum and

THE EAR.

expands as it proceeds downwards. This passes into the throat, and is known as the eustachian tube by which air is brought through the throat to the inner side of the drum, and permits the drum to vibrate freely.

People by swallowing can force air into it which is felt to crack in the ear; and when the throat is inflamed, the opening into it may be closed, and the sense of hearing greatly diminished.

The parts of the ear in which the sense of hearing is produced, are small, curiously and beautifully formed bony structures, known as the semicircular canals (Fig. 48), and the cochlea (Fig. 47) with which the drum is connected by a series of very small bones so connected together as to allow a little motion among them (Fig. 46). They are attached to two membranes, one at either end, and as the drum vibrates the vibrations are carried to the inner membrane, which sets in motion a very small quantity of fluid in the canals, and influences the nerve of hearing which is in contact with it.

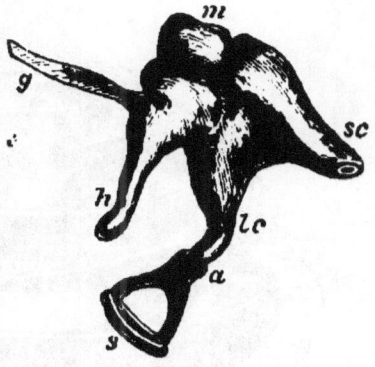

Fig. 46.
THE OSSICLES, OR LITTLE BONES OF THE EAR.

There are three bones, viz.—
s, The stapes, like a stirrup.
sc and ic, The incus, or anvil, like a double tooth.
m, The malleus, or hammer, with h, the handle by which it is attached to the drum (Fig. 45).

Hence the vibrations of the air are collected by the external ear, conveyed by the auditory tube to the drum, modified by the air entering from the throat, conveyed to the internal ear where they are perceived and the effect is carried on to the brain or mind by the auditory nerve. Sounds of all kinds and qualities can be distinguished by experience or special training, but their meaning is learnt by the sciences of speech and music and by observation. Vibrations of air, which are as slow as 16 and as quick as 24,000 in a second, can be heard. The slower the vibrations the lower the tone.

All these parts which in their healthy state assist in the sense of hearing may become diseased; and although in some conditions, as in inflammation of the brain and in certain nervous affections, the sense may be increased so as to be distressing, the common effect is to lessen the sensation of

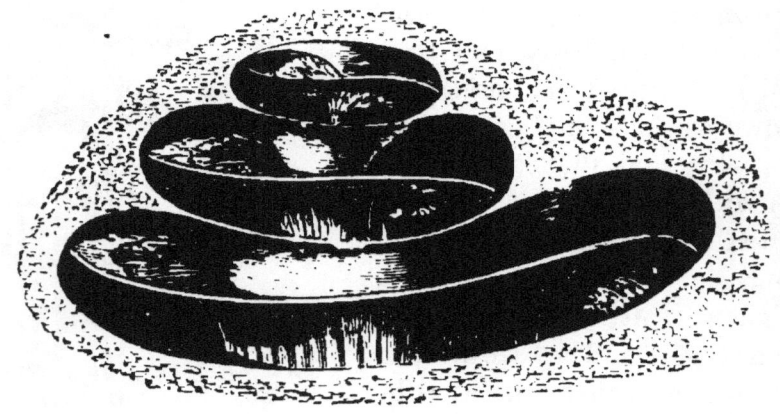

Fig. 47.

SECTION OF THE COCHLEA OF THE EAR.

This very beautiful structure resembles the interior of a snail's shell in form. There is a central pillar, which expands at the top, and around it a thin layer of bone winds in a spiral manner. The spiral cavity thus formed, is lined by very delicate structures, and is supplied with a branch of the nerve of hearing.

sound. This is produced by many causes, as thickening of the membrane of the external tube, too much wax, thickening of the membrane covering the drum, perforation of the drum, closing the eustachian tube, breaking the chain of little bones or ossicles, or diminishing their power of motion, and various diseases of the internal ear. Hence we have in the ear an organ which varies very much in its condition and fitness for hearing, and is influenced by a thousand external agencies as well as by the inevitable changes occurring in old age. Many children become deaf in early life, and nearly all persons are more or less hard of hearing in old age.

This is not the place in which to describe the diseases of the ear, but we may for a moment refer to two habits which

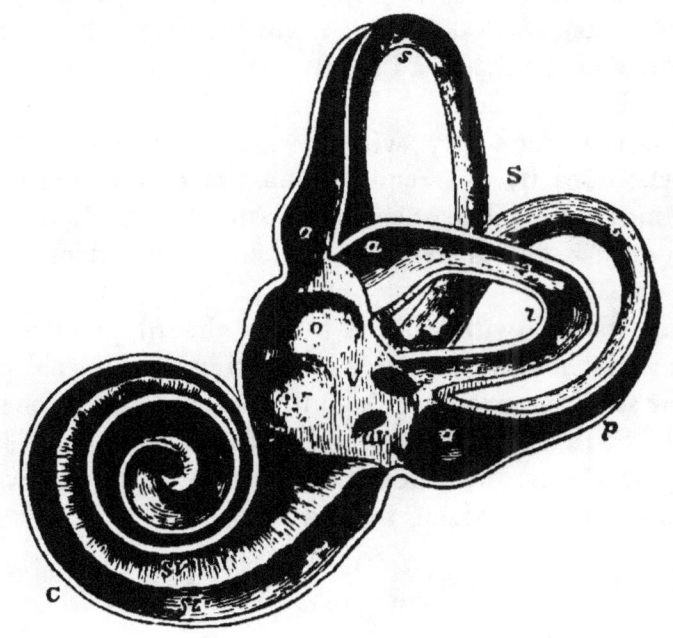

Fig. 48.
SECTION OF THE LABYRINTH OF THE EAR.

This remarkable bony structure in the ear consists of numerous parts, to which anatomists have given separate names, and is essential to the sense of hearing.
S, The three semi-circular canals.
C, The cochlea, of which an enlarged representation is given in Fig. 47.
V, The vestibule.

tend to injure this organ or to produce disease, viz., picking the ears and closing them with wool.

Picking the ear with the finger is exceedingly common in children, by which the skin on the inside is dirtied and irritated, and by causing it to be inflamed, produces a discharge. This again causes itching, and thereby tends to keep up the habit. In later life, a toothpick or a needle is used to clean out the ear, and irritates the skin the more, until by an accident it perforates the drum of the ear, and may permanently injure the organ for the performance of its duties. This is not unfrequently induced at first by the effects of measles or scarlet fever which set up inflammation in the ear, and then the bad habit steps in and the disease is perpetuated.

This occurs frequently without the knowledge of the person who does it, and requires the timely warning which a friend may give. No one should rub the inside or prick the ear or use any instrument which might perforate the drum.

Closing the ear with wool is a very absurd practice, and particularly in hot weather, and by making the internal parts of the ear sensitive prepares them to take cold and to become inflamed. Such a practice, if merely a habit, should be discontinued. If Nature intended the ear to be closed she would have made better provision for that purpose.

THE NOSE.

Many young children pick the nose, and cause sores which remain for years; and it is said that this is an evidence of worms in the bowels. The importance of the practice is not great, but it is desirable that a bad habit should be discontinued, and the cause removed.

STUTTERING.

The most important defect of speech is in that of stuttering, and its cause and remedy are but imperfectly understood.

It is not generally due to any known defect in the muscles or other parts by which speech is produced, but is probably owing to a defect of that nervous power which regulates the muscles, as to the order in which they should move. When a stutterer is excited, he stutters the more; whilst when he is alone, and forgets himself, he speaks more plainly.

Many persons profess to have methods by which this serious defect may be cured, and all that are rational are based upon the regulation of the acts of breathing and speaking. The first requirement is to induce the stammerer to take his breath in the usual regular manner, and not to hold it and emit it by jerks; and the second is to practise the speaking of all the vowels first, and then of all the letters of the alphabet slowly and perfectly. This will probably occupy twelve months, but with great watchfulness nearly every case may be cured. It is, however, more easy to effect this when the intelligence of the stammerer is enlisted in the process, and he is quite persuaded that it does not arise from physical defect, which is permanent, but from causes over which he has control.

CHAPTER XIII.

GENERAL REMARKS ON PERSONAL CONDUCT AND HEALTH.

We have now considered, in as much detail as the plan of this work permits, the leading subjects which are involved in the preservation of health and the prevention of disease, and it may be useful to sum up much that has been written in a chapter of a general character, and to add such remarks as have not found a place elsewhere.

The leading rules in the management of infants are to give as much warm milk as can be eaten, to allow as much sleep as possible, and to keep the body warm. After a few months of life, bread and farinaceous foods may be properly added, and in due time vegetables and gravy, bread and butter, and similar foods; whilst there may be much greater freedom of motion and exposure to the air allowed, and consequently somewhat less care in supplying external warmth.

It may be doubted whether meat is necessary to the health of a child under two years of age, but after that period it may be supplied in a very moderate quantity. Up to perhaps seven years of age but little more animal food than milk and eggs is required, provided that they can be obtained in sufficient abundance, but no objection can be taken to a very moderate supply of meat or soup. Broth should not form any considerable part of a child's dietary, since it contains very little nourishment. Fats are necessary, but if plenty of new milk be eaten there will be a sufficient supply, with the addition of butter to bread, as is the common practice in this country. If there be a dislike to fat meat, care should be taken to lessen it in a moderate and reasonable manner, but it will be unwise to *force* the child to eat it. A little coaxing, and the substitution of some kind of fat which is less disliked, will often overcome the difficulty.

The quantity of food eaten throughout childhood should be abundant, inasmuch as growth requires a large part to be laid up in the system, and probably not less than twice the quantity which would be given to an adult in proportion to weight, should be supplied up to fourteen years of age, whilst under one year of age it should be five or six times greater.

During all this period of life free exercise of every part of the body, free exposure to the ordinary temperature, and reasonable clothing should be supplied, so that the skin may not become too sensitive, the muscles may grow freely, and bodily agility may be acquired. If there should be feebleness of body there will be the more need for milk and meat, regulated exercise and moderate warmth.

At this, more than at any other period, it is desirable to follow a regulated plan of gymnastics or simple exercises, so that the body may be held erect and rest well on the hips, the legs lifted and thrown well forward in walking, the head erect, the chest open, and the shoulders thrown back—that is to say, those positions should be gained in which bodily exertion may be the most readily made, and the lungs have the freest action. Should the chest be flat and the shoulders round, or should the parents be asthmatical or consumptive, the greatest attention to these directions should be given. Posturing and exercises for ten minutes daily, by which the shoulders and arms may be thrown back, whilst the chest is expanded by deep inspirations, if begun in childhood, will probably suffice to prevent injury to health.

The period of youth and early manhood is that which usually determines the character, bodily and mental powers, and personal habits of the man, and is therefore fraught with his future fortunes. Sufficiency, without excess, of both animal and vegetable food; regulated hours of work, study, and exercise; avoidance of causes of debility, exhaustion and disease; daily habits of observation of natural and other objects; inquiries into the causes of things; due regard to the claims of relations and neighbours, and of our duty to God and man; a sense of responsibility tempered with a consciousness of seeking to discharge the duties of life faithfully, and to improve every faculty of body and mind, with due submission to the order of Providence and to those who are set over us, will tend to happiness, usefulness, long life, and health.

Early rising and a good breakfast are indispensable, with such exercise, study or labour, as we may be then required to make. Food before entering upon any continued or hard work; an early, sufficient, but not excessive dinner of meat, vegetables and pudding; a light tea and light supper, or a later and more nutritious tea, with reasonable variety of bodily and mental exertion and rest during the day, early retiring to rest, and sound sleep during seven or eight hours will tend to health.

If the person be inclined to be stout and wishes to become less so, he should not eat too much fat, bread, or farinaceous food; but prefer lean meat and skim milk, and yet take bread and fresh vegetables in moderation. Extreme means of this class may reduce the health as they reduce the fat; but the aim should be to improve the health, whilst more exercise and less food are taken. On the other hand to increase the tendency to lay up fat, it is necessary to eat new milk, fat and farinaceous foods as well as meat, and to somewhat lessen the amount of exertion, whilst the digestion and every function of the body are kept in their highest vigour. Thinness may not be an evil, and if it were, it may be due to a peculiarity of constitution which time alone can change; but at the period of growth and active exertion it is as natural, as is a tendency to lay up fat with advancing age and repose of mind or body. It is not unusually fat men who are the leaders in either bodily power or mental vigour and activity; and, as a rule, to lay up fat is to lessen mental action and clearness of mind. Whilst, therefore, a reasonable deposit of fat may be desired, any excess becomes a burden and a hinderance to the performance of duty.

If the object be to train for bodily work there should be regulated exercise of the whole body, as well as of that specially required, in a degree beyond what is ordinarily taken, whilst the diet should be almost exclusively of meat, bread, and fresh vegetables. Not more food should be taken than can be digested, nor more fluid drunk than the proper solution of the food may require. The aim must be to cause the greatest development of the muscles, and to supply abundant material for their maintenance, whilst all useless material is kept out or carried from the body. When training for running or rowing the diet consists of underdone and lean mutton-chops and beef-steaks, with a moderate quantity of bread and potato. Water is drank in a limited quantity, whilst all alcoholic liquors are rigorously excluded.

If the desire be to study with the greatest ease and clearness, the quantity of food should be somewhat restricted, so that a sense of oppression may not occur, while its quality should be that just described, with a further addition of milk, and perhaps of tea. With all this, the appetite, digestion, and excretions, must be kept in order by sufficient bodily exercise.

A word on the subject of fluids may be required here. The use of fluid is to soften the food and carry it into the blood; to remove from the body useless material, and to supply sufficient to the solid structures and fluids of the body. It is therefore necessary, but the quantity taken is usually more than is necessary. A habit of excessive drinking of any fluid is easily acquired, for the body retains or throws out fluid very much as it is supplied, and as some eighty to ninety per cent. of all the body (except the bones) is fluid, it is clear that bulk and weight may be increased by water alone. There is a power in the body both to fix and to discharge fluids from the structures in varying degrees. Hence it is an evil to drink too much fluid of any kind, and particularly water and tea; but the evil is less with the use of milk.

Fermented liquors should never be given to suckling mothers or to infants and children, except under medical advice, and as life advances the necessity for them in health does not increase, although they may be better tolerated.

These remarks are applicable to that very large part which is called middle life, during which all the powers of body and mind are developed, but it may be desirable to add a word on the subject of moderation.

Moderation in work and pleasure, in bodily exercise, mental labour and food, is the ground of health, usefulness, long life, and happiness. The whole object of life is not summed up in any one of these, neither should the accumulation of money be the end and aim of life. The present practice tends to excess of so-called pleasure by one and of anxiety by another class, both of which are unfriendly to the highest state of health, and are far less desirable than the simple application of the precept to "Provide things honest in the sight of all men," and "to do justice, love mercy, and walk humbly with our God."

In advanced life the special senses, as sight, hearing, and taste, lose much of their power. The bones are more rigid, the muscles weaker and less agile, all the vital functions languish, and everything indicates that the body as an instrument of power and work, is falling into decay. The mind also loses its force and activity, and with the subsidence of the passions a state of repose is, or should be, present, which gives, perhaps, as much pleasure as the stronger passions of earlier life could afford. Then appears the desirability of not having abused health, and of having made due provision for old age in a pecuniary sense, as also in the cultivation of the mind, which will remain when the cultivation of the bodily powers may have been lost. Happy old age without painful disease, with sufficient necessaries and comforts for the body, with a mind well stored, with resignation, without anxious thought, and with a good hope beyond the grave!

CHAPTER XIV.

THE SICK-ROOM.

It may not be out of place in concluding this work to add a few remarks which seem to advance beyond the region of health, and to enter the border-land of disease, for there are certain ailments, slight or frequent, to which persons in health are subject, who are yet said to be in health, and a few common and widely-spread conditions of suffering, which are yet, in the main, consistent with health. We do not profess that this is a very logical or clear distinction, but we think that some observations respecting them may be tolerated if useful.

A sick-room, whether used for a cold or other passing and temporary evil, or for long-continued disease, is not unusually hot, close, and dark—conditions the reverse of those which are required to maintain health. The doors and windows are carefully shut, the blinds lowered, and the curtains of the bed drawn as if the whole aim were to suffocate the patient. Generally speaking, the reverse of this should be found. The air should be fresh and sweet, which implies proper provision for the change of it; the fire should be moderate, so that the air be neither hot nor cold; the furniture should not be in excess, and no accumulation of clothes, whether clean or dirty, should be permitted. The carpet and floor should be scrupulously clean, and no accumulations of dust or dirt should be found under the bed or in corners. Every utensil should be perfectly clean, and emptied and scalded as frequently as may be necessary. White or coloured blinds and curtains, a few flowers, and other objects of interest, should be present, as well as such interesting books as may be obtainable and fitting.

The degree of quietness and darkness must depend upon the nature of the illness and the requirements of the moment; but, as a rule, the room should be made cheerful by the light, and the stillness should not be oppressive. Excessive sunlight and sun heat should be avoided, and needless tramping in and out of the room prevented; but the light of the sun, and the light of the human countenance do much to render a sick-room cheerful. Above all, let there be wise heads, willing hands, and loving hearts in the attendants, and thankful submission, with common sense, in the patient.

CONTAGIOUS DISEASES.

One of the most common uses of this room is for the ailments of children, which are of a contagious or infectious character, and which rarely occur more than once in life—such as measles and scarlet fever—the former of which is often so mild and unimportant as not to need the aid of the doctor, whilst the latter is often far more serious than it appears to be, and requires close attention and medical skill. More important diseases are produced by the neglect of proper precautions in the treatment of scarlet fever, even when it appears in the mildest form, than perhaps from any other ailment. Small-pox is the most important disease of this class, but it is, fortunately, disappearing.

In these, as in the more important contagious or infectious fevers, to which we do not propose here to refer, whether occurring at home or at school, it is perfectly necessary that the patient be kept quite apart from others for a certain time, in order to prevent the spreading of the disease; and, therefore, we may here give a few directions, which will be generally applicable.

1. The sick person should be rigidly restricted to one room or a part of the house which is separated from other inmates.

2. The room should be treated as already stated, and such disinfectants used as may be necessary. The best are Condy's red fluid, carbolic acid, and carbolate of lime, chloralum, solution of chloride of soda or lime, and chloride of lime. The fluids may be diluted and used by saturating cloths, to be hung in various parts of the room, and the chloride of lime by being placed with a little vinegar in a saucer. All these substances are poisonous, and should be carefully used, and, as the chlorine is irritating to the eyes, nose, and throat, it should not be too strong, nor used in all cases.

3. Disinfectants are, however, of little use as compared with fresh air, and therefore the first duty is to provide proper ventilation, without draughts or cold. The sense of smell is a good guide as to the state of the air, and, if the air be sweet, there is little for such disinfectants to do. The poison which causes the spread of the disease is greatly increased by concentration in close rooms, and decreased by dilution and free circulation of air.

4. The linen, clothing, bedding, utensils, and every object touched by, or in contact with the sick, should be carefully isolated, and such as will permit, thrown into boiling water, in which they should be well stirred and boiled for half-an-hour, after which they will be harmless. All others should be disinfected by other means.

5. The nurse should be restricted to the sick-room, or

otherwise isolated, and should not associate with any other inmates. All other persons, but particularly the children, when measles and scarlet fever are present, should not visit the sick-room, or touch anything used by the sick until it has been boiled, and, if possible, they should be removed from the house.

6. Remember that the disease is communicated by both the poisoned air about the sick, and by the clothes and other articles used or touched by them.

7. Measles may be communicated for a fortnight, and scarlet fever for six weeks after recovery, and during that time the child should not attend school.

8. Small-pox is a disease of too important a character to be discussed here, but in order to prevent it every person should be vaccinated, and, if necessary, re-vaccinated.

9. When the patient suffering from any of these contagious diseases leaves the room, the room should be disinfected.

This is best effected by boiling everything that will admit of it, by scalding, by scrubbing the floors and utensils, and by whitewashing the ceiling and walls, and it may be wise to take off the wall-paper. The room should be emptied if possible, and with the room and windows open for a day or two, admit plenty of air to every part of it. Chlorides may then be used freely, if they do not enter other rooms and cause irritation.

COLDS AND COUGH.

Another condition of universal occurrence is that of colds and coughs.

The name given indicates its nature and cause, for there is a marked sensation of cold, and it is usually induced by cold. The sensation is due to increased sensibility of the skin to heat only, so that with the ordinary temperature, the person feels cold, and yet the skin may be of its usual temperature. It is very common to see such an one sitting before a fire muffled up in every part, so that the external air cannot gain access under the clothing at the neck, wrists, or feet, and he even covers the parts which are usually bare, viz., his hands and head. He perceives the slightest movement of the air, and cannot tolerate any one moving near to him, lest currents in the air should be excited.

With all this the skin may be moist, or in its usual state, or somewhat dry, but with a cold merely there is not a state of fever, although it may be one of feverishness.

There may be sneezing, with discharge from the nose and eyes, if the cold appears like influenza; or there may be cough, with pains in the muscles, or coughing if it tend to bronchitis.

The cause is generally undue exposure to cold air without proper clothing and protection, but generally the air is also damp, as that of a valley or on a rainy day. Not unfrequently it is warm and damp; but then cold is obtained by throwing off clothing, sitting in an open window or door, or in a draught from some other cause, and thereby there is exposure of the body whilst the skin is unduly sensitive.

It may be asked why a current of air should give cold, when still air of the same temperature will not do so. This is owing to the fact that a larger quantity of heat is carried off when the air is in motion (assuming that the body is warmer than the air, as it is almost invariably in this climate), and therefore becomes cooler, although air in motion may not be cooler than still air. Hence, when we are too warm, we delight in a breeze, because it cools us; but if we are not too warm, or if we are too cold, we shun it, and the sensation of cold warns us of our danger.

There are some who sit in draughts carelessly, and take cold without knowing where and when; whilst others, almost by instinct, and without mental consciousness, avoid places where draughts are likely to occur, and sit in that part of the room which is not in the line of the door, window, and chimney. Hence the one takes cold frequently, and the other very rarely.

There are also some who have thin and very sensitive skins, which readily perspire, who are rarely without colds, whilst others have thicker and drier skins, and escape. Some are habitually careless about their dress, and make no provision for the occurrence of a shower, or a sudden change of temperature; whilst others wear thick shoes or boots, and flannel shirts, and carry a shawl or overcoat, and an umbrella under almost all circumstances. Which of the two is the wiser?

But one who is over careful may not be wisely careful, and by needless clothing may make his skin sensitive, and very likely to take cold; or so protects himself by staying at home in doubtful weather, that he fails to maintain good health. Some take shelter under a tree when there is lightning, which may strike the tree and kill him, or in a passage where the wind and rain rush along it, and he takes cold. Nay, even an umbrella may give cold if so held, that the wind is allowed to drive under it.

Again, the state of health predisposes to or protects against colds. One who is always sensitive, or recovering from an illness, or is specially liable to diseases which are brought on by cold, is unusually apt to take cold, whilst one in robust health, with the same degree of caution, is less liable to colds. Women, moreover, are perhaps more liable than men to this evil, although their duties less expose them to severe weather, because they are more sensitive, and less sufficiently clad, and, it may be added, are often forgetful of themselves in seeking to discharge their duties to others. Children and old people are also more liable than adults in the middle of life.

But in reference to all these special liabilities, it must be remarked that wise caution may avert danger, and unwise carelessness induce disease, and that in all cases it is a question of undue exposure to those conditions which give cold.

Exposure to very severe cold, as in a snow storm in Scotland, may produce extreme loss of heat, which goes beyond the idea of a cold, and the sensibility may be so benumbed that the person is not aware of his risk. This is also the case with very old persons, who are exposed to even moderate cold, and by which life may be brought into great danger.

Nature indicates the proper treatment in the outset of a cold by giving the sensation of cold, and the eager desire for warmth. To go to bed for two or three days, clad in flannel, but with not too much bed clothing, will give the requisite warmth, and take away the currents of air which give the sensation of cold; but the head, and hands, and neck should also be covered. To occupy a hot-air bath in which the air is both hot and dry, or a room having the same conditions, for twelve to thirty-six hours, will in the same way assist a cold, but a vapour bath will not have the same good effect, neither a room in which a fire gives an equal temperature. For such an one to sit directly before a hot fire, is to increase the disease, because the heat and the open chimney cause a great current of air towards the fire, and the person must be hot on one side and cold on the other. The true requirement is equal and sufficient warmth, without the least perceptible motion of the air.

Is it desirable to produce profuse perspiration? Not at the first, for perspiration further cools the body, whilst our aim is to warm it; but afterwards, with signs of feverishness, it may be desirable, not, however, to stop the cold, but to prevent fever. At that point the doctor is required.

Why are hot gruel and other hot fluids given? If given wisely, it is with a view to supply heat to the body and to stimulate the nerves, and therefore they should be as hot as the person can drink them. If they are given in too large a quantity they may produce great perspiration and be unnecessary if not prejudicial, and therefore they would not be wisely given.

Should food be discontinued during a cold? This is often decided by the patient himself, for he cannot eat; but to starve a cold, as it is called, is rarely wise. Ordinary but simple food, and that always hot and more than usually fluid, is the proper kind of diet.

Hence the golden rule is this: Do not sit in a draught, and when you feel cold take instant means to remove from the cause or to protect the body. With a cold, stay at home and keep the body warm from the first, and free from every atmospheric change. A cold which may be checked and cured in the first twenty-four hours, may be beyond reach of simple means, and assume far more important characters after the first day. Of nothing is the old adage so true that "a stitch in time saves nine." When you are in doubt as to the proper course, or not satisfied with the result, send for the doctor. Remember that colds are almost always preventible, and therefore should not occur, and when simple are almost always remediable, and should not be dangerous; but they do occur and do lead to great danger.

Bronchitis is now a fashionable name for a cold which affects the chest and causes cough. When applied in a strictly medical sense it is an important disease, but in the ordinary sense it is usually unimportant. A cold with an ordinary cough is called bronchitis, or a cough with some expectoration without other disease has the same designation, and particularly when the cough is severe and tight, and with some pain about the chest.

It occurs usually from a cold, and therefore under the conditions which give rise to a cold, as in the winter and in cold and wet seasons; or if in warm weather there has been undue exposure by sitting in draughts or without sufficient clothing or exposure to the night air. It will rarely if ever arise from dry cold unless there be an unusual tendency to the disease, as from previous attacks. The breathing of cold and damp air is very likely to produce it, but much more so if the skin be insufficiently clad.

Two-conditions exert a great influence over it, viz., the state of the throat and the skin. The act of coughing takes place in the throat, and whatever causes irritation there causes cough either directly or by the influence of the current of air over the throat as it passes down in respiration. One having an inflamed or very sensitive throat is aware that the current of air feels cold as it is inspired, when with the throat in its ordinary state no such sensation is experienced. Hence, whatever conditions make the throat inflamed cause cough, and such are among many, inspiring very cold air, drinking strong liquors, drinking or eating very hot things, smoking tobacco in excess, and inhaling charcoal or acid fumes.

The influence of the skin in producing cough is shown by the effect of a sudden chill, and it is chiefly through this part of the body that cold acts.

The act of coughing is a very useful tell-tale, established by nature to prevent improper substances passing down or remaining in the throat. Thus, if food enters the top of the windpipe instead of passing down to the stomach, a most violent cough is produced, with the intention of throwing it back and ejecting it from the mouth. If we breathe some injurious substance as coal gas, or the fumes from acid works, or hot steam, cough is excited, to make us aware of the danger. If there be too much secretion upon the throat or in the windpipe which would interfere with breathing, cough is produced, and it is dislodged and thrown into the mouth. It is not therefore correct to assume that cough is always an evil which should be remedied, for usually it is harmless or beneficial.

What then should be done with a cough?

1. If it has been produced by a cold, it should be treated as a part of the cold, and as the latter improves so will the former.

2. If there be much irritation in the throat, it should be treated in the throat by something which soothes that part of the body, as moderately warm and moist air, warm mucilaginous liquors as gruel, barley water, milk and water, and linseed tea, or by jelly, blancmange, jujubes, or liquorice, which dissolve slowly in the throat and by coating the surface protect it a little from the action of dry, cool, or irritating air.

In these applications it should be remembered that when the remedy has passed down the throat it is often of no further service, and therefore small quantities should be used and allowed to remain in the throat as long as possible before being swallowed. All stimulating substances as ardent spirits, pepper, vinegar, and pickles, by irritating the throat, increase cough, and should therefore be rigidly excluded from the dietary.

3. Do not attach too much importance to an ordinary

cough, but be content to use the ordinary means to remove it and to prevent its increase; but as cough arises from various diseases, both of short and long duration, if it continue long, or is severe, or occur without cold, or is accompanied by pains in the chest or by fever, apply to the doctor without further delay.

How many old persons are asthmatical and unable to enjoy life or to maintain themselves by their exertion!

Asthma is confirmed bronchitis accompanied by shortness of breathing and cough, and varying almost always with the weather. Nearly all such persons are ill during the winter and comparatively well during the summer, whilst a few are more afflicted in the hottest weather. The former are very sensitive to slight changes, but more particularly of damp and cold weather, whilst some can bear dry frosty air tolerably well. Hence the night is worse than the day, and sound sleep is not easily obtained. Nearly all such persons are liable to "attacks," and are not equally well in the same weather, and many are so affected that they are comparatively well in a house or a neighbourhood which would not be healthful to others. Each person has some peculiarity, and experience should be his guide.

With shortness of breathing it is not possible to run or to ascend stairs rapidly, or to make great exertion, as all such efforts require more breathing than can be made, and when the attack occurs the sufferer cannot lie down but must sit up in a chair or be propped up in bed. When the cough is very troublesome and the difficulty of breathing great the doctor must be consulted.

An asthmatic person should first be guided by his own experience as to the place and room in which to live, and the kind of diet and exertion suited to them, provided he have gained knowledge by experience. As a rule, the following directions will be proper.

COLDS AND COUGH.

1. He should avoid cold and damp air, and therefore wintry weather and exposure in the early morning or late at night.

2. If he can go to a warmer climate in the winter, he should do so.

3. A very damp climate or situation is almost always more injurious than a dry one; but yet a very elevated situation, exposed to strong northerly and easterly winds, is seldom fitting.

4. He should wear something like a respirator when he goes into cold air, so as to warm the air before he breathes it; but the ordinary respirator often hinders the air from passing through it, and he has to open his mouth and inhale the air around it. A muffler, or handkerchief, would often be more useful.

5. He should usually breathe through his nose, and keep his mouth shut, and thus warm the air as he inspires it.

6. When with exertion he is obliged to open his mouth to breathe, it is proper to consider whether the exertion is not too great for him.

7. His bedroom should be neither too cold nor too hot, and should be so ventilated that the air cannot be damp; and if the room be small, a fire should not burn during the night unless it be really necessary.

8. If sitting in a chair, or on the bed, the chest, shoulders, and neck should be covered with woollen clothing, lest he should take cold.

9. His diet should be simple and ordinary, and, above all things, the quantity of food or fluid to be taken at a time should be small, lest it should increase the shortness of breathing; and it should, therefore, be given frequently, and also in the night. Warm, and not cold, fluids and food should be given, and alcoholic stimulants are often injurious.

RHEUMATISM.

Rheumatism is the greatest plague of the working man, and yet is almost entirely due to man's neglect. The great soreness of the limbs and muscles, from which the shaking of a cough is intolerable, is of this nature, and if the cold could have been prevented, rheumatism would not have occurred. The rheumatic pains in the joints, which many have with damp weather, are due to improper exposure, and, probably, colds, in years gone by, which have left a tendency to renewed attacks; but they may also be due to local causes of suffering, as decayed teeth, and can be prevented only by the removal of the cause.

Rheumatism is, however, almost invariably due to cold and wet combined, and not to cold alone. Thus a fine frosty day may not induce it, if the body be properly clad, but a shower coming on, and the clothing becoming wet, even in a much warmer temperature, rheumatism follows.

Why do wet clothes give rheumatism? Because the water becomes converted into vapour on the skin by the warmth of the body, and by so doing causes cold, precisely as perspiration cools the body. If, therefore, the part in contact with the water were not too hot, it becomes too cold (although the other parts of the body may be warm enough), and thence produces rheumatism. Hence, when the whole body is equally wet, the probability is that a cold will be taken, and when only a part of it rheumatism may arise; or when, with the whole body wet, some part is dried and warmed, as by standing before a fire, whilst other parts may be wet and cold, the latter may become rheumatic.

Rheumatism differs from rheumatic fever in that the latter affects the whole body, and is accompanied by fever, whilst simple rheumatism affects particular parts, and there is no fever. Rheumatic fever is far more important than simple rheumatism, and may endanger life, whilst rheumatism causes much suffering, and often incapacitates the part affected for labour. But either, having once occurred, is liable to recur with even a much less cause than that which originated it.

Hence it is of great importance to avoid the circumstances which give rise to rheumatism, and to keep the clothing warm and dry. Should it become wet, do not dry it whilst wearing it, but change it. It is almost impossible to prevent rheumatism, and quite impossible to prevent its recurrence, in this climate, without wearing woollen clothing next the skin, and therefore the directions already given as to clothing should be attended to.

The treatment of an attack of rheumatism is not so simple as that of a cold, for it cannot be thrown off at once; neither can excess of heat be borne without increasing the pain. It is, however, quite essential to keep away cold and damp air from the part, and to cover it with woollen material, and very frequently increasing the heat of the skin by the application of heat as of a hot iron, or bag of hot water or salt, or by rubbing it, gives temporary relief. Other applications, of a medical character, are, however, usually required, such as stimulating oils, which act in the same manner when rubbed into the skin, with other remedies to directly relieve the pain; and the doctor must be applied to.

Whenever a child or young person has swollen joints which are tender to the touch, rheumatic fever should be feared, and the doctor sent for. Disease of a most important kind thus often commences in childhood, and shortens life.

HEADACHE, ETC.

Another very ordinary series of conditions may be classed together with constipation, cold feet and hands, and headache.

In order to maintain health it is well established that the bowels should be relieved once a day, and more is not usually necessary or desirable. This is commonly effected by the unassisted order of nature, but may be aided or retarded by habit and food. It is well to visit the closet at a fixed hour daily, and common experience shows that the hour after breakfast is the best. This habit should be regarded as one of the most important duties of life in relation to health, and nothing should be allowed to interfere with it. Food has also an influence; since green vegetables, and particularly those having acid juices, increase the tendency, whilst much bread has the contrary effect. Fats assist when they are eaten largely, and an unusual quantity and variety of food has the same influence. Spirits and alcoholic liquors have the contrary tendency.

It is desirable to distinguish between foods which aid naturally and those which act by causing irritation, since the latter may cause waste of food and set up disorder or disease. Thus brown bread causes relaxed bowels by the bran inducing irritation, and thereby nutrition is rather hindered than aided. Acid fruits and sour milk in summer act as medicines rather than as foods, and may produce too much action, and when they are indigestible, as pieces of raw fruit, may bring on serious diarrhœa. Whatever acts by causing irritation should be regarded as a medicine.

When there is a tendency to constipation due consideration should be given to the character of the food as well as to the habit above mentioned, and it will often be found that a glass of water or a seidlitz powder in water taken before breakfast, with or without a walk at the same time, will be a simple remedy. Due exertion is requisite for this as for every other condition of health, but excess in perspiration tends to produce constipation.

Cold hands and feet with only ordinary exposure show not only that the circulation of blood is defective but that the quantity of heat produced in the body is insufficient, and that the body should be kept warm. The natural mode of warming the body is to take food, but the appetite may be defective or the digestion out of order, and thereby the food is insufficient to produce the required effect. If this be due to ill health it must be remedied by other means, but warmth by clothing, fire, and hot food, by exertion and by rubbing the skin will be useful, and at the same time attempts should be made to improve the appetite and digestion.

No one should sleep with cold feet, but have a bottle of hot water in bed to remedy that evil. Hot milk is the best food.

Many suffer from intense headache which is not due to any apparent cause, but it usually occurs only when some function is out of order, and it is to such only that we now refer. With that condition the bowels may be constipated or the liver disordered. The appetite fails, indigestion occurs, cold hands, feet, and skin follow, and there is a general sense of languor and ill health. The spirits become low, and if there are troubles they are magnified, and we look at the dark instead of the bright side of the picture. Then the connection of mind and body becomes very apparent, and we are conscious that the former is by no means free.

Warmth to the body, warm food, a good aperient and perfect

rest in the lying posture, possibly in a still and dark room for some hours, and the evils sometimes suddenly pass away, and we see life again in its natural aspect. When this is not the result it is probable that the cause is deeper seated, and the advice of the doctor should be sought.

INDEX.

Ages, Personal conduct at different, 172.
Agricultural labourers, 77.
Alcohols not necessary, 54; waste of money in, 55.
Alum in bread, Test for, 19.
Arrowroot, 20; how prepared, 22.
Asthma, 188.
Atmosphere, Elements of, 136.
Atmospherical conditions, 136.
Auricle of the ear, 166; of the heart, 123.
Autumn, 146.

Bacon, 35; when cheap, 35.
Baking-powder, 18—20.
Barley meal, 15.
Barley, Pearl or Scotch, 20.
Bathing, 107; cold, 107; in sea, 108.
Beans, 16.
Beer, 53.
Bees should be kept, 8.
Beetroot, 5.
Black-puddings, 33.
Blood corpuscles, 126.
Blood-vessels, 124—128.
Board, Climbing, 91.
Bones, 32; cooked, 68.
Bran, 15.
Bread, 15—17; how made, 18; brown bread, 19; alum in bread, 19; cooking of, 67.
Breakfast, 174.
Breathing, 132.

Bronchitis, 185.
Brook water, 46.
Broth, 30.
Butter, 42.
Butter-milk, 42.

Cane Sugar, 6.
Carrots, 25.
Charcoal, Danger of, 114.
Cheese, 37; in South Wales and Wiltshire, 37; Stilton, &c., 37; in milk, 42.
Childhood, Food in, 172.
Circulation in man, 123; in frogs, 125; in plants, 126; variation in rapidity, 131.
Cleanliness, 104.
Climbing rope, pole, &c., 91.
Clothing, 70; for different ages and seasons, 72; at night, 72; travelling, 73.
Coal miners, 79.
Cochlea of the ear, 168.
Cocoa and chocolate, 52.
Coffee, 52; when to be preferred to tea, 52; action of, 52.
Cold baths, 107.
Colds and coughs, 181.
Condiments, 58.
Contagious diseases, 179.
Cooking, Hints about, 62; utensils to be clean, 63; ranges, 65; by gas, 65; waste by, 68.
Cooking of meat, 30.
Cowheel, 34.

INDEX.

Cornea of the eye, 158.
Cows allowed to feed in lanes, 42; should be kept, 43.

Damp course, 119.
Digestibility of many foods, 56; of cold food, 68.
Digestion, 122, 131.
Diseased meat, 29.
Diseases from occupation, 77.
Disinfectants, 180.
Disinfecting rooms, clothing, &c., 180.
Drains, 110.
Dripping, 30.

Ear, 164; outer and middle, 165; inner, 167; bony, 166—169.
Early rising, 174.
Earth closets, 111.
Eating raw meat, 32; diseases from, 33.
Eggs, 39; fried, 39; hard-boiled, 40.
Elements of the atmosphere, 136.
Electricity, 146.
Exertion, 74; effect of, 75; on circulation and respiration, 132; best time for, 76; at night, 76; by women, 76; violent, 77.
Eye, 155; diseased, 161.

Fat, 8; fat cells, 9; fat in many foods, 11; fat disliked, 12.
Fermented liquors to suckling women and children, 176.
Filters, 45; renovated, 45.
Fish, 38; dried, 38.
Flannel clothing, 73.
Flavour of cooked food, 67.
Flour, 14; adulterated, 16.
Fluid, how much, 176; use of, 176.
Foods, cooked, 62; warmed up, 68; where to be kept, 69; selection of, 122, 129; alike in kind of nourishment, 129.

Frog's foot, Circulation in, 125.
Fruit sugar, 6.
Frumenty, 20; how made in 1350, 20.

Gas, Explosions from, 115.
Gelatin, 34.
Giant stride, 90.
Golden syrup, 6.
Grinders, 77.
Gymnastics, 82; Mr. McLaren's school of, 83.

Ham, uncooked, 32.
Haricots, 17.
Headache, 192.
Health, Rules of, 153.
Heart, 33.
Heart, Circulation in, 123, 124
Heat produced, 132; regulated, 133.
Heat-producing foods, 5.
Honey, 7; poisonous, 8.
Horizontal pole, 85.
Horse chestnuts, 59.
Houses, 109; site of, 109.

Infants, Food for, 172.
Iris, 156.
Isinglass, 34.

Joints of meat, 31.

Labyrinth of the ear, 169.
Lens of the eye, 158.
Lentils, 16.
Light, 147; action of, 148.
Liquid foods, 41.
Liver, 33.
London and General Water-purifying Company's filter, 46.
Long sight, 159.
Lungs, 33.
Lungs, 127; of plants, 140.

Match-makers, 77.
Meals 129.

INDEX.

Meat, 28 ; character of good, 29 ; uncooked, 33.
Milk, 41 ; for infants, 41 ; cold, 41 ; diseased, 43.
Millers, 77.
Mind, and mental work, 150 ; effect on health, 151.
M'Laren's system of gymnastics, 83.
Moisture in the atmosphere, 143.
Monkshood root, 60
Mountain-ash berries, 59.
Muscular fibre, 28.
Mushrooms, 59.
Mustard, 58.

Nettles, 23.
Night, Circulation and respiration in, 132.
Nightshade berries, 59.
Nitrogen in air, 137.
Norwegian-stove, 66.
Nose, 170.

Oatmeal, 14 ; requires much cooking, 15 ; cakes, 19.
Occupation, 77 ; in close rooms, 77 ; the effects of, 77 ; remedies against, 78.
Offal, 33.
Oil, 9 ; in cocoa nut, 10 ; in milk, 10.
Open fire, 114.
Ophthalmia in schools, 161 ; causes of, 161 ; remedies for, 163.
Ossicles of the ear, 167.
Oxygen in air, 136.

Parallel poles, 87.
Parsnips, 25.
Passover-cakes, 20.
Peas, 16.
Pease-pudding, 17.
Pepper, 58.
Personal conduct and health, 172.
Perspiration, 105.
Petroleum, 116.
Petties, 111.

Physiology, Sketch of, 120.
Pickles, 59.
Pigsty, 111.
Plumbers, 77.
Poisonous substances, 59.
Pole climbing, 90.
Pork, 28.
Potato, 23 ; quantity eaten daily, 23 ; cooking of, 24 ; when cheap, 24 ; diseased, 24, 25, 26 ; berry of, 59.
Poultry and game, 36.
Pressure of the atmosphere, 142 ; effect of, on body, 142.
Puff-balls, 59.
Pulse, 17.

Recreation, 80.
Rest, 95 ; on Sunday, 99.
Rheumatism, 77, 79, 190.
Rice, 20.
Rope climbing, 90.
Rye meal, 15.

Sago, 20 : how obtained, 21.
Salt, how much required, 58.
Salting meat, 31.
Sausages, 29 ; diseased, 33.
School-room, its ventilation, 162.
Season, Effects of, 145.
Shops, Unhealthy, 80.
Short sight, 159.
Sick-room, 178.
Silber's lamps, 116.
Skimmed milk, 42.
Skin, Section of, 134.
Sleep, 100 ; by day, 101 ; best in early night, 101 ; conditions of, 101 ; how many hours, 102.
Soils for site of houses, 110.
Sound, rate of travelling, 147.
Soup, 30, 33.
Spinach, 23.
Spirits, 53.
Spring, 146.
Squinting, 160.
Starch, 12 ; starch cells, 13 ; starch in foods, 14.

INDEX.

Stomata of plants, 140.
Stoves, 113.
Stuttering, 170.
Sugar, 5; sugar-cane, 5; sugar-maple, 5; sugar in foods, 7.
Sweat-glands and pores, 134.

Tailors, 80.
Tapioca, 20.
Tea, 48; proportion of weight and bulk, 49: how to make it, 49; adulterated, 50; scarcely a food, 51; not fit for children, 51.
Tobacco, 60; injurious and wasteful, 61; preparation of, 62.
Treacle, 5.
Trichina spiralis in flesh, 33.
Tripe, 34.
Turnip-tops, 23; turnips, 25.
Typhoid fever from milk, 43.

Veal, 28.
Vegetables, Fresh, 23.
Ventilation, 116; of workshops, 79; of houses, 116; bedrooms, 117; of schools, 162; of pantry and cellar, 118.
Ventricles of the heart, 123.
Veronica, 60.
Vinegar, 59.

Warmth, 112; by stoves, 113.
Water, Foul, added to milk, 43.
Water, in many foods, 44; filters, 45; hard, 47; cool, 47; deficient in villages, 48.
Water-parsley, 60.
Weekly rest required, 98.
Week's work, Effect of, 98.
Well, 111.
Wet clothes, 79, 190.
Whey, 42.
Windpipe, 128.
Wines, 53.
Wooden horses, 92.
Woollen clothing, 70.
Workshops, Unhealthy, 80.
Worms in flesh, 33.

Yeast, 16; yeast cells, 16.
Youth, Food in, 174.

THE END.

www.ingramcontent.com/pod-product-compliance
Lightning Source LLC
Chambersburg PA
CBHW020903230426
43666CB00008B/1289